HOW TO USE A FORK

ORLANDO SWAYNE

HOW TO USE A FORK

STORIES OF MENDING THE BROKEN BRAIN

PICADOR

First published 2026 by Picador
an imprint of Pan Macmillan
The Smithson, 6 Briset Street, London EC1M 5NR
EU representative: Macmillan Publishers Ireland Ltd, 1st Floor,
The Liffey Trust Centre, 117–126 Sheriff Street Upper,
Dublin 1 D01 YC43
Associated companies throughout the world

ISBN 978-1-0350-6433-5 HB
ISBN 978-1-0350-6435-9 TPB

1 3 5 7 9 8 6 4 2

A CIP catalogue record for this book is available from the British Library.

Typeset in Perpetua Std by Palimpsest Book Production Ltd, Falkirk, Stirlingshire
Printed and bound in the UK using 100% Renewable Electricity by CPI Group (UK) Ltd

MIX
Paper | Supporting responsible forestry
FSC® C116313
FSC www.fsc.org

To Delia, Madeleine and Sol

A NOTE ON THE TEXT

The events in this book are based upon my experiences in clinical practice. Details of both patients and colleagues have been used with permission or altered, and some people about whom I write are presented as composites. The book is intended for the general reader and does not in any way constitute medical advice.

CONTENTS

PROLOGUE

The hospital where I work sits proudly in the corner of a Georgian square in London, a Victorian carbuncle resplendent in showy red brick. Like many hospitals of its period it has a chapel, Anglican and reasonably high church, complete with shiny marble floor, altar cloth and stained-glass windows. This is an oasis of quiet tucked away at the centre of a busy hospital like the secret eye of a storm. If you poke your head in you will often find a nurse sitting quietly having just finished their shift, or a hospital porter leaning forward on a prayer mat. Sometimes when nobody is about I will sneak in for a few minutes to find my calm centre in the middle of a busy day.

This occasion was different. I was tucked into a row of chairs along with ten or so of my colleagues from the neurorehabilitation unit, sitting quietly as we were led through a short service. This is more remarkable than it sounds. The minister leading the prayers was at that time one of our inpatients.

A lean man in his mid-fifties, Thomas was a busy vicar working across two home county parishes. He was married with teenage children, had a quiet intensity in conversation and a doctorate in history. Seven long months previously he had collapsed in the middle of a service, with a spontaneous bleed into the base of his brain that rendered him unconscious. Thomas spent around two months on intensive care and awoke from his coma as the blood gradually cleared away, but in the process had suffered damage to several important structures at the bottom of his brain.

Only months before this service he had needed support for all his bodily functions: a tracheostomy tube in his neck for breathing, another tube in his stomach for feeding, and another in his bladder. Even now he had double vision, almost incomprehensible speech, poor balance and difficulty moving or feeling his right side. Until recently he had been unable to sit up in bed, much less stand.

After months in rehabilitation spent grinding through the nuts and bolts of basic life skills, Thomas had insisted on making his next goal something that was meaningful to him. So there we sat on our chairs, listening while he stood and read aloud from the Book of Common Prayer. Without an ounce of irony, he of all things gave thanks.

We were transfixed. As a congregation we were a motley group, all staff from the rehab unit who worked with Thomas. To my right sat our psychiatrist Himanshu, then our charge nurse Dennis, a junior doctor, a couple of other nurses and some uniformed therapists. Put this team in a room together and you would usually hear rustling patient lists and conversations flying in all directions. Today nobody moved as we watched Thomas take charge of the chapel, transformed from the patient in Bay 3 Bed 1 into the master of his realm.

As he stood in front of his wheelchair Thomas held tightly onto the frame before him. One therapist crouched to his left and supported his pelvis from the side, while another held the text out in front of him close enough to read. One eye was covered with a patch. The familiar sacred phrases burst out into the chapel like bullets from a Gatling gun, staccato, disjointed and difficult to resolve at first, but no less impassioned for their lack of smoothness.

Thomas fought his way determinedly through the text, sweat

beading on his brow from the effort. As his words engulfed us everything else seemed to recede – the distant sounds of the hospital, the support needed for him to stand there, even his illness – leaving just one man and his willpower. You do not need religious belief, it turns out, for the hairs on your neck to stand up in a chapel.

How was Thomas able to do this? He had bled from an artery into his pons, a region that sits right in the middle of the brainstem, as the brain's base is known. Mention of the brainstem will cause your typical student of anatomy to break out in a sweat. It is densely packed with scores of nerves and tracts, criss-crossing like an oddly symmetrical railway map. Some connect the brain to the eyes, ears, nose and tongue, while others control blood pressure and organs such as the heart. Being so full of vital anatomy, the brainstem is particularly sensitive to damage – tiger country to a neurosurgeon brave enough to venture into it – and damage there often causes severe and permanent disability.

Given the site and extent of Thomas's brain injury, then, conventional thinking would rule out what we were witnessing in the chapel. Such a scene should be impossible or highly unlikely. Yet there he stood.

*

Over the past twenty years a quiet revolution in neuroscience has been changing our perspectives of the brain, how it responds to stroke and other injuries, and what this should mean for how we think about rehabilitation and recovery. Once, a patient like Thomas would have been written off as beyond help and destined for nursing home care. In this book, I will explain how new insights into what happens when the most complex organisational system in the known universe (the human brain, not the National Health Service) becomes damaged – and especially into the crucial role played by the subtle process known as neuroplasticity – have enabled us to get Thomas and others like him back to a semblance of their previous lives. This shift in thinking has profound implications for what we should believe is possible, and also perhaps for the treatment and care that we owe such patients.

Our brains are organic super-computers: billions of nerve cells with trillions of connections between them, all in constant chattering electrical communication. Within the patterns and flickering traces of these connections dwells our entire conscious being: our innermost thoughts, profound and profane, our hopes, fears and memories. Here in this ghostly framework also live the skills we need to interact with the world, to stand and walk, to play the piano or type on a keyboard, to speak, to laugh. If a brain area is damaged then these traces and connections vanish. There is an immediate loss of function corresponding to the region involved.

As a student I was taught that the brain does not mend. Once an area becomes damaged, we were told, that is it. You might see a little improvement over the first few weeks as things settle down, but there is little to be done that will affect the outcome. As a result of this orthodoxy such patients received relatively little attention once the immediate medical issues had been taken care of. Traditionally, if you were brought in with a stroke the doctor would prescribe bed rest, nurses would take care of your bodily functions, and you would be shielded from stimulation or activity. As will become clear, every aspect of this approach is precisely the opposite of what we now know is needed.

It is perhaps easy to see how this nihilistic approach came about. At the level of a standard microscope, neurons – the brain's nerve cells – do not regenerate once injured. Neurons in mammals are relatively unusual in that they do not reproduce at all once mature. A fully grown adult has pretty much all the brain cells they will ever have and, unlike skin or the liver, a damaged area will never grow back.

This may seem at first glance like an evolutionary misstep: in most vertebrates, such as fish or amphibians, a damaged nerve cell will simply regrow. In fact, this capacity has un-evolved in several independent branches of the evolutionary tree: the neurons of mammals and most birds are actively prevented from regenerating by the surrounding cells. So this change must presumably confer some advantage, and it is interesting to speculate as to what that may be. Some suggest that it reduces the brain's vulnerability to the growth of tumours or the spread of infections. Others believe that this represents an evolutionary trade-off to maintain the stability of such a highly complex structure. The long-term memories that mammals and birds are able to maintain are held in fine balance for years within their brains' structures: this feat would seem difficult if new neurons kept popping up across the network. Perhaps the price the brain has paid for such stability is an incapacity for regeneration.

With the circuits responsible for a particular function wiped out by a stroke or other injury, then, one might reasonably expect the loss of function to be permanent. If my MacBook's graphics card packed up I would not expect it to mend itself spontaneously. This is a belief that has found its way into the general consciousness, and which still pervades among doctors and medical textbooks. But it turns out not to be the whole truth.

Other changes take place within the brain after injury, changes that are more subtle and extraordinary than simple regrowth. Surviving brain tissue undergoes extensive reorganisation, forging new connections and creating new networks over time. The term neuroplasticity describes a fundamental feature of the brain whereby it is shaped by its experience of the world around it. It has been described as a subtle but orchestrated dance between the brain and the environment, allowing us to learn new skills and to make ever truer internal models of the world we inhabit. If harnessed, this may allow functions to be restored that were thought to be lost. Because there is no obvious change at the structural level – little to see under a microscope – this process of reorganisation is hard to perceive and measure. Its results, however, may be dramatic and its implications for how we should manage recovery are profound.

This change of perspective has been gradual, for myself and for the wider neuroscience community. Having been told that brain injuries were irrevocable I began as a junior doctor to meet patients for whom this was clearly not the case. Something was changing in their brains that enabled a degree of recovery. Over the last twenty years there has been an explosion of investigation into neuroplasticity, using ever more sophisticated methods to shed new light on our brain's response to change or injury.

Our brains' neurons speak to each other via their synapses – the electrochemical connections between one neuron and its neighbours – and it is within these that the magic of neuroplasticity is found. Among the thick mesh of cells the synapses connecting adjacent neurons allow pathways to form, chains of neurons that are connected in sequence like an invisible route through a dense jungle. With an estimated hundred trillion synapses – each individually adjustable – the branching complexity of the brain's circuits is almost unimaginable, and it is here that the capacity for reorganisation resides. Neuroscience has over recent years shed much light on how this works, revealing plenty that is startling and beautiful. Watching this story unfold has been like taking a microscope to the underside of a leaf only to find a hidden city.

Neuroplasticity is fundamental to how our brains learn. Information about the world around us leaves its trace in our neural pathways and is retained. With trillions of synapses being adjusted in real time our brains' models of the world around us are constantly being moulded, our lived experience and personal history encoded in innumerable tiny synaptic clefts.

One of the ways that our brain makes sense of the world is by maintaining strict spatial relationships between its cellular circuits and the corresponding body parts they are controlling, or the aspects of the world they are encountering: adjacent circuits are laid out like maps of the body or outside world. The fluidity of these neural representations that synaptic plasticity enables is central to the story of this book and to the experiences of patients like Thomas. It allows reorganisation to take place in response to a change in circumstances in ways that we can now measure or see. Regions adjacent to the damage may be brought into play in a re-moulding of networks, with latent connections linking distant areas opened up for use. What is more, we seem for a while to enter a hyper-plastic state resembling that seen in a young developing brain.

The idea that synaptic plasticity drives recovery after an injury is no idle curiosity – it opens up all sorts of possibilities. We know from experimental work that we can influence neuroplasticity in a variety of ways, so can we do the same for patients? This question has given rise to a wide field of enquiry and has led neuroscientists to develop ever more outlandish ways of kick-starting recovery from stroke and brain injury: from medications, to electromagnets, to chips in the brain, to virtual dolphins (of which more later).

Most importantly though, this new field of research tells us increasingly clearly that intensive and high-dose therapy and training are what drive recovery. This allows potential gains such as the recovery of lost speech, improving memory or concentration, or new movement in a weak limb – these in turn may translate into invaluable improvements in independence and quality of life. I am privileged to witness this process every day.

*

Clinical practice has in many cases struggled to keep up with the science. An outdated view pervades which sees neurorehabilitation as a field lacking real treatments, a dowdy poor relative of sexier branches of medicine in which new molecular or cellular treatments are revolutionising outcomes. Within the fields of stroke and brain injury, resources tend to be concentrated at the more acute end of the pipeline with less consideration given to the journey to recovery that follows. But it is this journey and how it is managed that largely determines where that person will end up: passively dependent on the care of others or capable of self-determination. Sequestered from society or actively engaged with those around them.

Too often those with stroke leave hospital without adequate provision for rehab, denying them the chance of a meaningful recovery. The situation for head injury is even worse. Almost universally patients are sent home once they can walk and talk, with little regard for the major changes in thinking skills that often occur. Failure to address this invisible disability sets up patients for years of struggling to regain their lives, and often also leads them into trouble.

It does not have to be this way. If you were to consider rehabilitation as a medication, with a dose you can vary and an effect you can measure, we would all be buying shares in the company that made it. The extent of its effect on quality of life puts to shame most drug trials that make it to national press. It is now clear that the previous conservative approach has condemned generations of people with brain injuries to accept poor outcomes. This needs to change. We would not accept poor availability of antibiotics for chest infections, nor of aspirin for heart attacks – why are we OK with poor access to rehabilitation after brain injury?

My relationship with the human brain has altered dramatically since as a child I first wondered how it worked. It continues to evolve now as a neurologist, as each week I am astonished by some new capability. I have been taught lessons in neuroplasticity by long nights trawling the wards as a junior doctor, by working with brain-injured people, by practising the piano and by observing my children. My eyes have been opened to how much a good team can achieve in transforming somebody's prospects, and to the gap between what is often accepted and what is possible. The journeys of these patients also take us at times to the edge of the human experience and back again, as a person's being is reconstructed one circuit at a time.

In the stories of those struggling to fight their way back to a semblance of their previous self we catch a glimpse of the human determination to continue to exist in the face of catastrophe. This book is therefore a testament not only to the brain's extraordinary capacities but also to the indomitable force that resides within people and their families – a force that allows them to get back up again after being struck down by neurological injury.

Far from lying dormant, as previously assumed, the injured brain is constantly finding new pathways and forging new connections like the restless roots and tendrils of an apparently peaceful garden. New shoots will emerge, but they need tending and nurturing if they are to take. Our challenge is to work with this force and harness it to its full potential – to begin putting the pieces back together.

CHAPTER ONE

THE MAN WHO LOST HIS LEFT SIDE

We had a new patient on our ward. Christian was a gentle and softly spoken man of nearly seventy. With a sparkle in his eye and a raffish shock of black hair he brought to mind a Filipino Marlon Brando. Before his recent stroke he had worked as a 'mixologist' in the bar of an expensive London hotel.

Before going to meet him, I spoke to his wife Julie. I found her standing by the nurses' station asking about visiting times, so I introduced myself. As we talked a call bell was going off in the next patient bay, a nurse was in conversation with the ward pharmacist, and wheelchairs were approaching from either direction. Builders had just started work on what was to be a quick refurb of Bay 4 and one of them had a radio on. I suggested that we escape the ward's bustle, so we moved up to the day room – high ceilings, sunlight streaming in through tall Victorian windows – and found a table in the corner.

Julie was petite with quick bird-like movements and short black hair tucked behind her ears. The strain of recent weeks showed in the crinkles around her tired eyes. She sank back into a red padded chair, and as she absorbed the relative calm of the day room she uncoiled slightly. I asked her about the events that had led to this point, but she brushed aside my medical questions and told me about Christian the man.

'Doctor, have you been to smart cocktail bars before?'

I admitted that I might have done, once or twice.

'Making cocktails is usually a young person's game, not for old people like Christian and me. But he is funny and charming – everybody loves him at the hotel. Christian is the kindest person I ever met, always ready to help somebody if they need it.'

She leaned in and gripped my hand.

'He is everything to me. I need him back, and I am relying on you.'

When I met him, Christian was lying diagonally across a bed, unable to right himself. A hospital gown was caught awkwardly round his shoulder and gaped a little below. His left arm and leg were like dead weights, ignored and jammed up against the side of the bed. It was apparent from where I stood that he could not see or feel anything on the left side, as if the canvas of his world had been torn vertically down the middle and one half discarded. Lying beached on the bed, he seemed as comfortable as a fish on a riverbank.

As I looked at Christian I tried to imagine how I must seem from his perspective: half a person perhaps, peering down at him from a distorted world. I moved over to his better right side, perching on the hospital bed. I asked him how he was feeling today. Could he tell me why he was in hospital? He made no answer but grabbed tightly onto my wrist with his right hand. He fixed me with a desperate look from which I gathered that he could not understand a word I was saying.

I tried leaning in and speaking louder (traditionally the preserve of the Englishman abroad). Corrugated blue paper curtains were drawn around his bed in a farcical token of privacy. I tried again.

'When did you get here, Christian?'

Ron in the next bed piped up, his rasping East London tones cutting through the flimsy curtain.

''E's been 'ere since yesterday, doc. Can't 'ear a thing.'

I kept going, struggling now to maintain the pretence of separate cubicles.

'Are you in any pain?'

Ron again.

'Honest doc, 'e's deaf as a post. Doesn't seem in pain though.'

Our charge nurse Dennis was next to me, a kind and gentle presence in his dark blue uniform. He tried asking the same questions again in Christian's native Tagalog. But Christian just held onto my wrist and looked back and forth between Dennis and myself, as if appealing for something we could not give him.

The junior doctor fetched a whiteboard and I wrote the same questions out. Christian peered closely and it seemed he could now understand them, but when he took hold of the pen and scrawled out four words they read 'I love my wife'. After this he was overcome by the effort and sank hopelessly back onto the bed.

This was not going to be an easy conversation for him.

A stroke is a sudden loss of function in part of the brain resulting from an interrupted blood supply. It is the single largest cause of disability in adults worldwide, and in the UK alone racks up billions each year in the costs of healthcare, long-term dependency and loss of economic activity. Around ten years ago the annual cost of stroke in the US was estimated at $34 billion and it is expected to triple over coming decades. Stroke also ruins lives.

The brain plays host to our thoughts, our skills and our entire lived experience through its three-dimensional gossamer-like network, a near infinity of connections held for years in delicate balance. A stroke cuts a terrible swathe through our conscious being, eradicating skills and knowledge like a fire sweeping through an ancient library. The story of neuroplasticity and its potential benefits starts for me with stroke: being the most common form of brain injury its effect on our lives is the greatest, and the challenge it sets for those seeking to promote recovery the steepest.

*

It had been the weekend, and Christian was out shopping with his wife. They had got up early and made the journey to one of the Essex suburbs to use the shops there. They were planning a trip to visit family in the Philippines and were after some presents to take with them.

At around noon he was pushing a trolley along the aisle of a discount shop when he became aware of a dizzy feeling. He ignored it at first, but after a few seconds his vision seemed to blur and his left leg began to give way. He called out to Julie but she did not hear, and his outstretched arm brought a cascade of chocolate boxes down upon him as he sank to the floor. At this point the shopkeeper noticed and they rallied round, but it was clear that something was seriously wrong. Christian lay prone but, try as they might, they could not sit him up. They asked him what was happening but he just groaned in response.

Julie had some nursing experience. She knew that it was important to get him to a hospital, and fast. Paramedics were called: as he could not move one side they suspected a stroke, so he was whisked under cover of blue light to the nearest stroke centre. As the streets flashed by, Christian was silent and clung tightly to Julie with his right arm, while his left hung uselessly at his side. She felt numb. After a lifetime's adventure together, and a journey that had taken them across the world, she was terrified that he was dying.

When a patient arrives in the emergency department of a stroke centre there is a whirl of activity that may appear chaotic but is in fact pretty organised. Since 2010 the immediate treatment of stroke in and around London (described scarily as 'hyperacute') has been concentrated into a handful of stroke centres. The aim is to start specialist treatment as soon as possible after symptom onset, and this centralised approach has since been shown to have saved many lives.

Hyperacute stroke treatment has been described, not entirely fairly, as glorified plumbing. A major stroke typically occurs when one of the brain's larger arteries becomes blocked, and the region that has lost its blood supply simply stops working. The symptoms that herald the stroke depend upon the part of the brain involved, but often include weakness on one side of the body.

The aim of hyperacute treatment is to unblock the artery, restore blood flow, and so save as much brain tissue as possible. A series of large studies have shown consistently that the quicker you do this the better the outcome: time is brain, and the first minutes and hours are crucial.

A sudden blockage in a large artery is often caused by a blood clot, which either may form at a tight narrowing or travel in the bloodstream from another part of the body altogether, becoming wedged as the arteries enter the brain and become narrower. The quickest way to remove a clot is to dissolve it using medication given via a drip. This practice, known as thrombolysis, came into widespread use in the late 1990s and transformed immediate stroke treatment. The drug is a synthetic version of a natural enzyme, which switches on another enzyme called plasmin: this in turn acts as a molecular pair of scissors and chops up the fibrin which holds the clot together.

In a best-case scenario the blocked artery opens up right away, the blood flows back into the stricken region, and the patient will magically transform before your eyes: moving the affected side, or becoming more alert and beginning to speak. It is hard not to experience a bit of a God complex when this happens and the patient sits up Lazarus-like before your eyes, though in reality the effect is rarely that dramatic.

As Christian's ambulance swooshed him into the hospital's emergency department the stroke team were waiting for him. He lay immobile on a trolley in the resuscitation room, surrounded by monitors and oxygen cylinders. Under the harsh lights the doctors in scrubs checked him over. He was in some distress and found it hard to comply fully with being examined.

'Christian, lift up your arms.' No response. They lifted both arms for him and demonstrated keeping them in the air. The right remained in position but the left flopped down again. It was the same story with his legs, and they noted that he was not moving the left side of his body at all. His head and eyes were turned firmly over towards his right side. He seemed unable to see anything coming towards him from the left, or to feel a pinch given to his arm or leg on that side.

The clinical diagnosis was clear-cut: stroke.

*

For as long as I can remember I have been aware that the brain is the seat of who we are. I spent a lot of time as a child reading comics. My favourite strip was The Numskulls in *The Beezer*, which illustrated this idea in graphic form: teams of little people lived behind the eyelids of 'Our Man' and controlled his body. Brainy (bald with glasses) lived at the top and made most decisions. Blinky pulled levers behind Our Man's eyelids and Luggy was in the Ear Department. Snitch hung around the nostrils, a large clothes-peg clamped to his own nose. They would all scurry about, exchanging telegrams with other Numskulls further down the body. Our Man lived with his aunt and did not seem to get up to much, but he was good at getting into scrapes. Sometimes Numskulls from other creatures would climb in through his ears, and he would start running about like a dog or flapping his arms like a pigeon. *The Usborne Book of Knowledge* – a wonderful and much-thumbed colourful compendium – went a stage further.

Scores of tiny people occupied a range of departments inside the head and throughout the body, all performing different functions. There was even a library in the brain, with bookshelves labelled 'previous experiences'.

This was an attractive idea for a young me, and I am sure played a role in what I do now. Conversely the idea of damage to this precious centre always held a particular horror in my mind. Family legend was rife with examples. 'Mad Jack' Benett, one of my grandfather's predecessors, had returned altered from a series of distant wars. He kept thumbscrews on his desk as macabre souvenirs – of what exactly, nobody would ask. Prone to rages, he was pacified with the same copy of *The Times*, freshly ironed for him each morning before breakfast. As they put it in those days, it was generally understood that he was 'not quite right'.

There was also my mother's cousin, who was very dear to everyone and a fixture at family gatherings. A largely silent presence in the corner of the room, she would sit impassively for hours with a mask-like face, listing over to one side and chain-smoking. She seldom spoke, but when she did it was with a loud and slow drawling monotone that would cut like a chainsaw through the general chatter. Out of the blue she would pose the questions that others might be pondering but would never ask. A cousin's new girlfriend would all of a sudden be fixed with a gimlet eye and asked 'Have you had sex yet?' or 'Do you have a lot of money?' while I sat wide-eyed, wondering what she would say next. Her conversational grenades made Christmas a lot more interesting.

Before my grandfather's funeral in my teens I had been warned that one of the cousins I would meet there was 'a little unusual'. After the service we all stood packed into the kitchen of a Wiltshire cottage, clutching glasses of the wine that my grandfather had picked out in advance for the occasion. When I finally met the cousin in question he seemed bright as a button to me. He chatted away cheerily with an infectious smile – refreshing in the circumstances – and I could not understand what the fuss was about. Then he said breezily and without the slightest hint of malice, 'It was so nice to meet your stepmother. I would very much like to have her stuffed.' I forget my reply.

It was clear that there was something different in how these relatives' brains were working. The thoughts and information they were processing did not somehow seem to be coming out in the usual way. I could imagine their Numskulls running about in disarray, dropping their telegrams and tripping over their laces.

Later in my teens, one of my mother's closest friends, Jenny, had a large stroke in her forties. With one half of her body heavy like a lump of concrete she was unable to stand and was slow to speak: hard to reconcile with the exuberant person we had all known growing up. Jenny was the matriarch of a loud and endlessly entertaining family, with five children and an exciting house that we would escape to from London at weekends. To a child in drab late seventies England her household seemed dizzyingly glamorous, an oasis of anarchic fun where anything seemed possible. We played Murder in the Dark and watched videos. They had American cereals, and even a waffle machine. Suddenly, and at a young age, Jenny was dependent on others, and after an initial spell in hospital she went to live in a care home.

When my mother first went to visit Jenny she took as a present a large ornamental brassica plant, signifying her new status as a cabbage. This pretty sick joke reflected the sledgehammer wit that these two old friends shared, but also the prevailing view of the time: stroke was irrecoverable.

My perspective on the apparently unmendable brain would change but not as a result of anything I learned at medical school, where the old dogma still held sway. Even an esteemed neurologist at the National Hospital at around that time scoffed at the very idea of neurorehabilitation as a discipline, asking how many ways there were to give someone a walking stick.

The shift in my thinking would take years of learning from patients and colleagues.

Jenny had the last laugh. With relish, she reminded me of the ghoulish present at my mother's funeral.

*

We are wired up back-to-front, with each half of the brain controlling the opposite side of the body. From Christian's immobile left side the doctors assessing him could therefore be confident that the stroke would be on the right, most likely due to a blockage of one of the brain's four main arteries. His new irregular heartbeat, picked up on that first examination, meant that the likely cause was a blood clot moving up from his heart to his brain.

Even though the likely diagnosis was pretty clear, you cannot in this situation just give the thrombolysis medication without first doing a brain scan, for one crucial reason. In about 15 per cent of cases a stroke is caused not by a blockage but by a bleed from an artery into the brain's substance, a so-called haemorrhagic stroke. Thrombolysis in such a situation would massively worsen the bleed, potentially with dire consequences, and it is essential first to rule this out. The 'door-to-needle' time is audited nationally, and the crucial medication is often started while the patient is still in the scanner in order to chivvy things along.

Christian was wheeled on his trolley into the CT scanner, the manic bustle of the emergency department replaced by an eerie sterile calm as he lay on the table inside the large doughnut-shaped machine. Behind the scanner's window the stroke doctor peered at the images of Christian's brain as one by one they appeared on the screen.

There was no sign of bleeding. There was subtle patchy darkening of the brain substance within the right hemisphere, suggesting the early effects of a cut-off blood supply. A special scanning sequence was then done to map out the blood flow in the arteries themselves. This confirmed a complete blockage of one of the main arteries on the right.

Even with a standard blocked artery stroke there is a small chance that giving thrombolysis medication might provoke a bleed into the affected area. This can happen anyway, as the newly damaged brain tissue is fragile, but thrombolysis makes this rather more likely. The longer you wait the more susceptible the brain becomes to bleeding, and the lower the chance of reopening the artery. So there is a strict time window for thrombolysis, currently four and a half hours since symptom onset, and a scary balancing act of risks versus benefits. Even with this risk, though, the chance of the medication reopening the artery means that overall, the odds are in your favour. In other words, as long as it does not cause a potentially fatal bleed, then it will probably help.

After the doctors spoke to a stunned and frightened Julie about potential risks, Christian received the thrombolysis medication. He did not deteriorate, but he did not improve either. He remained inert on the left and turned towards the right: thrombolysis had not reopened the artery.

Anybody who has called Dyno-Rod for a blocked drain knows that if pouring chemicals down the loo has not worked then it is time to start poking things around the U-bend. We have witnessed over recent years a further revolution in acute stroke care: the introduction of 'mechanical thrombectomy', or clot retrieval.

Another frightening conversation about potential risks – this time of stripping off the artery's lining and causing another stroke – and another trip on his trolley to the radiology department. The noise of the emergency department fell away once again as Christian was brought into the angiography suite, dimly lit and populated by masked figures in large lead aprons. He was brought alongside a table and slid across onto it, where the mask-wearer-in-chief began to clean an area of skin on the right side of his groin. He asked Christian to lie as still as he could, and to try to ignore what he was doing.

The radiologist numbed the skin at the top of one leg with local anaesthetic and then fed a long wire into Christian's femoral artery, peering through his glasses at a monitor suspended from the ceiling. He pushed a button and around Christian an enormous machine sprang to life: two X-ray units each the shape and heft of a cartoon anvil, joined by an eight-foot semi-circular hoop with his head at its centre. This apparatus whirred as it spun back and forth, the metal slab passing inches from Christian's nose as it worked to get the best possible view of his arteries.

Guided by this machine the radiologist fed the wire upwards into Christian's heart and out the other side, heading north up the internal carotid artery in the neck and toward the base of his brain: the site of the blockage. A tiny clot retrieval device was then deployed, fed all the way up the guide wire and used to scoop out the two obstructing clots. A fiddly version of the wire loop buzzer game, with supercharged consequences. The radiologist chatted away idly as he worked, the reassuring small talk belying the fact that he was rootling around with the blood supply to a live brain. Christian gave no response to the chat and lay apparently frozen with his eyes fixed on the ceiling.

The aim with all acute stroke treatments that seek to unblock the artery is to save brain tissue which is compromised but not yet irretrievably damaged. It is only worth attempting thrombectomy in some cases of stroke. The clot must be obstructing one of the larger arteries in order to be retrievable, and there must still be some salvageable brain in the affected territory. This tissue under threat is often described as the 'penumbra', like the edge of a shadow. The ideal candidate for such treatments would have a small infarct (meaning established stroke) at the core of the artery's territory, like a peach stone, and a large salvageable penumbra around the outside, like the flesh of the peach.

In the early to mid-2010s a series of large trials showed unequivocal benefit of thrombectomy in patients who were eligible. Almost double had a good outcome versus thrombolysis alone, with no difference in complications.

For Christian the procedure went ahead without incident, and the blood flow in the arteries as they appeared on the screens seemed to be improved, but there was again no discernible improvement in his clinical state. As he was wheeled out of the angio suite he remained as impaired as he had been before the procedure.

Julie followed along the corridors behind Christian's trolley as he was moved up to the hospital's acute stroke unit, a ward on one of the upper floors. As they climbed slowly in the lift he gripped her wrist with his strong right hand as if his life depended on it.

Arriving on his new ward, Christian was set up in the corner of a six-bedded bay. To Julie this looked like any other ward, but here appearances were deceptive: this was a stroke unit, a dedicated ward where early post-stroke care is highly protocolled. The staff nurse on his bay spent a good half hour checking him over and working her way systematically through a stroke care plan. He was hydrated via a drip. His blood pressure was kept in the right range with medication. His blood sugar was monitored. He was turned regularly to prevent pressure sores. She assessed his ability to swallow and found that he could not do this safely, so she inserted a feeding tube via his nose into his stomach.

Within an hour of landing on the ward Christian was seen by a physiotherapist and an occupational therapist, or OT. The physio worked on the physical aspects of his stroke such as his position in the bed. The OT, trained to dissect what makes a task difficult and fix it, looked at his basic self-care. They tried to get him moving, avoiding as much as possible the secondary complications of immobility. His neurological status was monitored for any deterioration that might suggest a change in the stroke. He was comforted and reassured by nurses who are used to looking after patients in this state.

The rolling-out of stroke units was underway around the time that I was doing my medical training in the 1990s and was really the first major revolution in stroke care. Previously, a patient like Christian would be put in a general medical ward, next to patients being treated for pneumonia, asthma or bleeding stomach ulcers. The rough rule of thumb was that after stroke around a third of patients would not survive, a third would live with disability, and a third would recover well. This has changed, and the improvement relates largely to stroke units. Patients in the weeks following a stroke are sitting ducks for infection, pressure sores and blood clots. Without specialist nursing, regular therapy input and stroke protocols they would fester and develop any number of complications. Swallow checks would be missed and they would succumb to pneumonia, a common killer after stroke, as food goes down the wrong pipe into the lungs. Simply by organising the care of stroke patients into dedicated units, stroke mortality in the UK was reduced by over a quarter.

Before long the medical team rolled into Christian's bay. In front came a clean-shaven man with an earnest smile, checked shirt sleeves rolled up and smart loafers. He introduced himself to Julie as Dr Aston and told her that he was the stroke consultant, though to her he seemed improbably young. Behind him trailed a woman who seemed even younger and who Julie presumed was the junior doctor. She appeared to be physically attached to a computer on a trolley, and as she pushed this along she thumbed distractedly through a patient list with one hand.

Dr Aston spent a few minutes asking questions, examining Christian as best he could and flicking through scans on the computer. As he concluded he turned to Julie and let a pause settle over her before he spoke.

'Your husband has had a significant stroke, I'm afraid. As you know we've tried to open up the artery but we haven't seen a great deal of change. We'll see how things go over the next few hours, and we'll repeat a CT scan either this afternoon or tomorrow.'

'Thank you, doctor. But what is the treatment now?' Julie's voice was small and she could feel her stomach shrinking.

'We need to do some further tests to find out what caused the stroke, and we'll start him on some new medications.'

As the ward round moved on out of the bay Julie sat numbly on the chair by Christian's bed. She held his hand and stared into space. A slightly acrid smell of fish rolled down the ward towards them as staff started to serve lunch to the first bay. Julie felt helpless and horrified. Was that it?

There is often a moment in such situations when the patient and their family realise that no further surgical or other specific treatments are planned. After the quick-fire pace of early events – fear of immediate loss, rapid decisions about treatment options and desperate waits for the outcome – there is suddenly no rush at all, for it seems that there is nothing more to be offered. For the patient's family, having been sustained on adrenaline and fear there is a lull in activity, and the frightening realisation dawns that this damaged state is in fact the new status quo.

Christian could not safely sit up and needed all of his bodily functions seeing to. The prospect of ever getting him home seemed remote indeed.

So it was that around five weeks after his stroke Christian was transferred to our neurorehabilitation unit to embark on the next phase of his journey. Our job was to make sense of the neurological damage, to optimise conditions for recovery and to use intensive therapy to drive the process. The aim was to reassemble the pieces of someone who until only recently had been Christian, and to enable him to live with a degree of independence and autonomy that would be tolerable.

The scale of the task was daunting. He had not sat in a chair for over a month, and when our physiotherapist Katie came to see him it was clear why. With another colleague she tried to sit Christian up on the edge of the bed. They propped him between them but he lurched immediately over to the left, his overactive right leg pushing down hard into the floor. He clasped onto Katie with his right hand but just could not find his upright, so they laid him carefully down again. He was going to need equipment to sit out.

Katie fetched an adapted chair which tilts back, with supports on either side and a head rest, and she brought it alongside. They worked a large sling underneath him, connected it to a hook mounted on the ceiling and hoisted him upwards. As Christian dangled over the bed and the electric motor whirred he called out, 'Julie, Julie!' His wife was not there, and he seemed to be in pain from his left side, but as Katie lowered him into the tilting chair he settled down.

They positioned him as best they could, and although he was only half upright he was at least straight and in no obvious pain. Christian looked about him and flashed Katie a twinkly smile.

'Thank you,' he said. 'Now I can see what mischief you are getting up to!'

And, as staff and patients came and went past his bay, he could now give them a nod and say hello.

We took a look at his immobile left arm. It was held semi-flexed at the elbow, wrist and knuckles. Christian winced when we touched it, even a light brush of the skin seeming painful. The arm was stiff. I gently stretched it out, having to pull against resistance which increased if I moved too quickly. Slowly, Katie and I were able to bring Christian's arm into a straight position. To prevent the muscles and tendons from shortening with lack of movement he would need regular stretching, medication for the hypersensitivity and the stiffness, and custom-made splints for the elbow and wrist.

We brought Christian's bedside table in front of him, cluttered with the remnants of breakfast, grapes from his wife and untouched magazines. He was turned slightly towards his preferred right and seemed not to notice anything on the left side of the table. Katie asked him if he would like a cup of tea – we had found that if you almost shouted into his right ear he could just about make you out – and he nodded enthusiastically. This was fetched but because of his dodgy swallow the nurse in his bay had to add thickener to it, a powder that renders a hot drink into a sludge rather like wallpaper paste.

Christian was clearly happy to be upright and able to see what was going on around him, but gradually the imbalance in his limbs began to twist him leftwards in the chair. He showed a slowly mounting restlessness, fidgeting and shuffling about. He waved his arm at the nurse in the bay, and when she came over said, 'Toilet, please!' He could clearly feel it coming but could not stop it, and soon it was too late. He was hoisted painstakingly back into his bed for a pad change, but by then he appeared too wiped out to focus on what Katie was trying to do. Defeated, he sank back on the bed and lay across it at a jaunty angle, his ignored left arm caught in the cot sides.

This was the start of a long slog. Seeing Christian lying across the bed, dependent and stranded, it was hard to know where to start. The sense of loss of his pre-stroke self, as the gentle barman with a sparkle, main earner and family man, was almost complete.

*

Faced with such overwhelming disability, we start by trying to break down and understand the impairments and how these relate to the anatomy of the injury. We listed Christian's impairments and, decoded from medical jargon, they were as follows. Left-sided weakness, with overactivity of the strong right side (so-called pusher syndrome). Some spasticity (muscle over-activity) in the left arm. Altered sensation throughout the left side. Loss of vision in the left visual fields of both eyes. Hemispatial neglect of the left side of space (more of this later). Impaired hearing. A cognitive communication disorder. Reduced attention with distractibility. Pain in the left shoulder and left knee. Intermittent agitation and distress.

One issue at least was solved early on: his apparent difficulty understanding speech. I got rather carried away, and tentatively diagnosed central deafness due to stroke in the temporal auditory processing regions: this is pretty rare, and usually only occurs when both sides are affected. In fact this problem largely resolved when we had him fitted with a new hearing aid. So I had to row back from 'unilateral cortical deafness' to common-or-garden deafness. I lost my fancy diagnosis but we could at least now hold some sort of conversation.

All of Christian's impairments could be related to the site of his stroke, a moderately-sized area of by now established damage within the right frontal, parietal and temporal lobes. Surprisingly, these affected areas all sit within the territory of one large artery.

Four arteries running up the neck provide all of the brain's blood supply: the carotids at the front and the vertebrals at the back (left and right for both). You can feel the carotids pulsing away if you put your fingers just to one side of your Adam's apple and press gently. This is the artery that detectives check in films when they find a body on the floor, before saying 'he's gone'. It takes freshly oxygenated blood up from the heart towards the brain, snaking its way through the base of the skull and emerging about two inches behind the eye.

The vertebral arteries at the back cannot be felt in the neck, as they are encased in the bones of the spinal column. Once they pass through the topmost vertebra (called Atlas after the Greek demi-god: like him it carries the weight of a large globe on its shoulders) they loop through the bottom of the skull and pop out at the base of the brain at the back, where they join into one chunky basilar artery in the middle.

With two internal carotids at the front and one large basilar at the back, evolution could reasonably have patted itself on the back and left it at that. Instead, it does something rather clever: all these arteries join up via small communicating branches, so that a circular loop is formed. This is the circle of Willis, and it resembles a small necklace sitting just underneath the brain's base. Heading upwards from this circle are the three large cerebral arteries on either side – anterior, middle and posterior – that feed the brain's hemispheres.

This arrangement allows for a degree of redundancy: if one of the four large neck arteries gradually narrows there is still scope for blood to flow through the circle of Willis and continue upwards. If a cerebral artery becomes blocked, however, there is no alternative supply, and then you have a problem. When Christian collapsed in the discount shop it was because this had happened to the middle cerebral artery (the MCA) on his right side.

The brain itself consists of a smallish brainstem at the bottom, sitting above the spinal cord near the back of the skull, on top of which sits a plum-sized structure on either side called the thalamus, and on top of that the enormous domes of the two cerebral hemispheres. To give an idea of size, the brainstem is about three inches long whereas the hemispheres span the length and breadth of the skull's top half and make up almost 90 per cent of the brain's weight. Each gyrus, or fold, is half an inch or so across, and it is these which give the hemispheres their walnut-like appearance. Sitting just behind the brainstem and tucked beneath the cerebral hemispheres at the back is a smallish structure called the cerebellum (little brain), which is important in the accurate control of movement and in some aspects of learning.

The brainstem is tightly packed with circuitry vital to the smooth running of our bodily functions and to getting information in and out of our brains. The large cerebral hemispheres on top are where most of this information is processed, and they do almost everything else. For convenience they are separated anatomically into lobes: frontal, temporal, parietal and occipital. From these hemispheres originates almost all of the brain's ultimate output – movement and language. They also process all input – sensation from the body, smell, sound and vision.

The cerebral hemispheres provide the mystical link between input and output and determine how one gives rise to the other according to its many internal processes – memory, reason, personality and abstract thought – all of which lurk within the brain's estimated hundred trillion or so connections.

I have always enjoyed the thought that every animal is in essence an elaborate input-output system, turning the information we receive about the world around us into a behavioural response. The ultimate aim is the same: to get food in one end of our digestive tract (and presumably out of the other). With expanding nervous systems evolution has simply found increasingly sophisticated ways of doing this, from the nerves controlling the wriggling motion of a worm as it filters its way through the soil to the brains devising leveraged derivatives to squeeze more out of the financial markets. We humans pride ourselves on our capacity for reason – although a quick glance at the news is usually enough to cure me of this fallacy – and this is reflected anatomically in our massively outsized frontal lobes compared to other animals.

Unluckily for Christian, of the brain's three cerebral arteries the MCA supplies the greatest part of the hemispheres, about two thirds. Relatively modest areas at the front and back are supplied by the anterior and posterior cerebral arteries, and the crucial brainstem is fed from small branches that come directly off the vertebral and basilar arteries below.

When the MCA becomes blocked, the proportion of its territory that is affected depends upon how far along the artery the obstruction forms. In a worst-case scenario, with a clot at its origin, the entire MCA territory may be lost. If a smaller clot finds its way further along the artery then it may obstruct one of the smaller branches, taking out only a proportion of the territory. The further along the obstruction, the smaller the stroke.

The resulting symptoms depend entirely on the regions affected. The brain's many functions are not distributed evenly but are organised topographically – laid out like a map – with each region performing specific roles. The idea that brain functions are localised to individual regions has been around for years but was developed in detail by neurologists in the Victorian era. David Ferrier and John Hughlings Jackson, both based at the National Hospital in London, used clinical observations and experiments with animals to produce a basic map for the control of movement in different parts of the body.

Ferrier would expose the surface of a dog's brain and apply an electrical current at differing positions. One would make a paw twitch, while another moved a leg. (Ferrier was in fact the first person ever to be tried under the Cruelty to Animals Act for his efforts.) With the advent of increasingly sophisticated brain imaging techniques there has been an explosion of human brain mapping, and these days you would need satnav to find your way around. Many functions are performed by networks of these brain regions but can broadly be attributed to particular areas.

Christian had lost a lot of important capabilities. Given the amount of brain machinery housed within its territory it is not surprising that a complete MCA stroke of either side is a devastating event.

For each of its functions relating to the outside world – controlling limb movements, processing sensations from the body, interpreting visual information – the brain's surface houses maps where its representations are laid out. You can find movement maps in the frontal lobe, sensory maps in the parietal lobe, visual maps in the occipital lobe and so on. Looking closely reveals several of each, hierarchically arranged and representing different aspects of that function.

When it comes to these spatially arranged functions the brain is largely symmetrical, so a complete MCA stroke will cause a number of deficits affecting the opposite side. There will be a loss of movement (the leg may be relatively spared, as its representation lies within a neighbouring artery's territory) and altered sensation. There may be difficulty paying attention to anything on that side. There may be visual loss from that side of space. An imbalance in eye movement control may mean that the patient's gaze is pushed to one side, seemingly looking away from the stricken half of their body.

For functions which do not lend themselves to spatial organisation, however, the symmetry breaks down, and the two hemispheres perform entirely different roles. The most important example is language, which is represented largely on the left side of the brain (known as the dominant hemisphere) in almost all right-handed and most left-handed people. A complete left MCA stroke causes a loss of language, or aphasia, which is probably the most devastating deficit of all. The left side is also responsible for reading, writing, verbal memory and calculations with numbers, all of which may be affected by stroke on that side.

Conversely, a complete right MCA stroke will spare language but cause other deficits: navigation or spatial awareness, the ability to recognise faces, or to interpret other people's expression of emotion, visual memory. A stroke in a smaller branch will result in loss of some of these functions but not others.

Christian ticked all of the boxes for a complete right MCA stroke.

It is helpful to us as we work with patients like Christian if they and their families understand something of how the changes they see have come about. So about a week into his stay I brought Christian out of the ward in his wheelchair and into one of our clinical rooms, airy and sparsely laid out for such meetings: a benched desk, a computer and some chairs. We exchanged information. Julie told me more about Christian's background, and of his likes and dislikes (sweet Filipino pastries and Justin Bieber respectively). I went through the brain scans with them and explained what the damaged areas they could see on the screen usually do. I also explained that while we cannot make these areas grow back we can encourage the remaining brain tissue to reorganise, and that this helps recovery.

Julie was engaged and attentive, and she maintained gentle encouragements to Christian throughout, but she looked tired. This usually (I suspected) elegant woman of a certain age was getting through the day in yesterday's tracksuit bottoms and a T-shirt, and the lack of sleep showed. Christian was able to take in about half of what I was explaining, sometimes leaning forward and peering at the scans with interest but at other times sinking back in his wheelchair as the weariness kicked in. We managed about half an hour before he ran out of steam, and one of the nurses came to fetch him back to the ward. As Christian was wheeled away Julie thanked me for my time and for everything that we were doing. Then she took both of my hands in hers and leaned towards me.

'Doctor, I need to know: will I get my husband back?'

There is not a simple answer to this question. In the lull

between the initial rush of treatments and the admission to our unit almost five weeks later a lot of hope and expectation had come to rest on what we would be able to achieve with Christian. The one question that Julie understandably wanted answered was impossible to address meaningfully at that stage: by how much would he recover?

You can have a rough idea of what to expect based on the history so far, the current clinical state and the brain scans, and in relation to some specific aspects you can be quite accurate. It would be unwise, though, to make a confident prediction at that point about his overall state. The only way to gauge how much independence Christian would regain would be to observe his response to therapy over the coming period – given the extent of his impairments at that point his prospects did not look very promising. But this would not have been a helpful speculation to voice to Julie at that point, and I explained that we would know more within a few weeks. I told her that he would certainly be changed from how he was before the stroke, but that we would help him to live the best life he could with his symptoms. This seemed scant comfort.

*

Many patients used not to survive a complete MCA occlusion. The fall in mortality is due in part to stroke units but also more recently to the wider use of an operation called decompressive hemicraniectomy. When an area of brain tissue loses its blood supply the dying brain cells disintegrate and the beautifully organised cellular structure gradually becomes an amorphous mush. Large protein molecules leak into the tissues, and fluid from the blood vessels follows by osmosis causing a chain reaction of swelling, like around a badly sprained ankle.

If the stroke is relatively small then such swelling does not matter too much, but after a complete MCA stroke this is potentially a major problem. The brain sits within a confined space, and while the skull is very good at protecting it from injury it is unforgiving when it comes to an expanding brain. The result is downward pressure on the vital brainstem, which is squished against the skull's base in a process known as 'coning'. This often comes on gradually two or three days after the stroke, and the patient becomes progressively drowsier.

Left untreated this would usually be a fatal development, with a mortality of around 80 per cent, and is known pessimistically as 'malignant MCA syndrome'. Older patients are relatively protected from this by virtue of having smaller brains (sorry, but it is true – our brains start to shrink from our mid-thirties onwards). If it is picked up early then a disastrous outcome can be avoided by involving a neurosurgeon and asking them to perform a decompressive hemicraniectomy. This involves taking off part of the skull on the affected side, usually about the size of a side plate, and closing up the scalp again but without the bone. This results in a very lop-sided appearance but saves the patient's life.

Some months down the line, all being well, the swelling will have gone down again and the 'bone flap' can be put back. Sometimes this is temporarily stored inside the abdomen and I have had more than one patient ask me some months down the line what the mystifying hard lump is in their tummy. Alternatively, a titanium plate is printed to fit the defect and repair the skull.

When hemicraniectomies began to be performed there was concern that this would result in more patients surviving with severe disability and a poor quality of life, so it was often reserved for right-sided stroke (when language is not involved). Subsequent studies suggested however that in fact many patients did better than expected, and a good proportion of patients on our rehab unit now arrive with almost half of their skull missing.

*

When we first assessed him, Christian's situation seemed desperate – he was in considerable distress and needed two trained nurses working together to manage his basic needs. Julie was herself nearing seventy and it seemed inconceivable then that someone with such high care needs could be looked after at home. He seemed destined for a nursing home. What chance would we have of changing that outcome? The brain does not regrow. A stroke or other injury leaves a permanent scar of dead tissue in the affected region. A swathe of Christian's Numskulls had effectively been wiped out in a freak accident, so where was any recovery to come from? Equally, with a damaged brainstem, how would Thomas, the stricken yet determined vicar, ever achieve his aim to work with parishioners again? In fact, as we will later discover, the processes of neuroplasticity and reorganisation led both people down different paths from those we would first have imagined for them. But I do wonder: if the methods that we now use had been available to Jenny in the 1990s, and to others like her, would their prospects for recovery have been different?

CHAPTER TWO

UNPICKING KNOTS

Priya's brain was under attack, though she did not know it. She was sixteen, a healthy sociable teenager who had just finished her school exams and broken up for the summer. The long break stretched before her, with its promise of weeks spent with friends doing everything and nothing. She was working evening shifts in a local pub, saving up to go to a festival in the Isle of Wight. The summer was her oyster.

That Sunday Priya had a headache and her parents, Dayan and Karen, noticed that she was acting a little strangely. She had a slightly childlike way about her speech, and when she surfaced from her room in the mid-morning she put on a Peppa Pig DVD. She started pre-announcing what she was about to do: 'I am going to sit on the sofa.' As the day went on her parents noticed that she made occasional odd movements with her arms, as if she were stroking a cat.

That evening Priya's sister Geetha returned from visiting her boyfriend abroad. She had received some odd text messages from Priya over the weekend and was worried. That evening Priya suddenly cried for no obvious reason. She had been late back from her friend's house the previous night – her family thought that an early night was in order.

The following morning, however, brought no reassurance. Priya did not emerge at all and when Karen knocked on her bedroom door there was no answer. Karen let herself in to find the room in darkness, so she headed for the window to draw the blinds. As she quietly made her way across the gloom she glanced up and her heart jumped. Priya was sitting on the edge of her bed in the dark staring straight ahead.

Karen let in the light and took her daughter's hand.

'Priya, love, are you OK? What are you doing?'

Priya mumbled inaudibly and her lips quivered slightly but she was unable to reply and seemed barely aware of her mother's presence. Karen called Dayan to come quickly. Priya's arms made small writhing movements that came and went. She would reach out towards an invisible target or seem to look at something that was not there. By now her parents were seriously worried and they took her in to their local hospital's emergency department. It would be over a week from this point until a correct diagnosis would be made.

The attack on Priya's brain was insidious and from within. There was nothing so crude at play as a blocked artery, but rather a diffuse and sophisticated infiltration by her own immune system – more a cyber-attack than an artillery bombardment. Priya's white blood cells had gone rogue and were churning out antibodies directed against one of her own proteins, the NMDA receptors on the surface of her brain's neurons. Once antibodies latch onto their target they trigger a cascade of immune attack systems – as a special ops soldier on the ground might 'paint' a target for an air strike – and unleash inflammatory havoc.

We are used to seeing inflammation of our skin: the red angry appearance around a cut that has become infected, or an area of sunburn. When the inflamed tissue is brain then it is called encephalitis and, as you might imagine, the consequences can be grave.

The NMDA receptors under attack are not spread evenly across the brain but are found especially in the limbic system, a rim-like swirl of structures near the brain's centre which is involved in memory and emotion. This form of 'limbic encephalitis' typically starts with emotional disturbances and odd behaviour. People might develop insomnia and rush about manically, or they might be lethargic or even paranoid about those around them. As it progresses this often leads to more clear-cut psychiatric symptoms such as hallucinations, then abnormal repetitive movements, epileptic seizures and eventually coma.

Dayan explained what had happened to the triage nurse. The Covid-19 pandemic was in full swing and everybody in the department was gowned, gloved and masked. The nurse told him that one of the doctors would see Priya soon, but that he would not be able to remain with her while she waited. Dayan implored her: Priya was not well, and she needed her mum and dad. The triage nurse was firm.

'I'm sorry, love, you'll have to wait outside.'

Dayan and Karen retreated and sat miserably in their car for three hours, not knowing what was happening and imagining the worst. Once they were eventually allowed in, masked and gowned, they found Priya sitting alone in a curtained cubicle while a nurse watched from outside. She was not speaking at all and looked bedraggled. Her pigtails had come loose so that her wavy hair sat straggled across her forehead. There were streaks of saliva around her mouth. She was by turns agitated and catatonic, with a restlessness that would ebb and flow. She sat cross-legged on the trolley, rocking back and forth, then got up and paced about. She made a range of odd movements with her limbs, such as rhythmically opening and closing both hands in time with her eyes. At other times she would stiffen all over and her eyes would roll back into her head. I have seen several young patients in this stage of NMDA receptor encephalitis, and it is hard to watch. Even once a diagnosis is made the level of agitated distress can bring to mind a scene from *The Exorcist*.

Unsurprisingly, by now Dayan and Karen were terrified. They had no idea what had happened to their daughter and so far it seemed that nobody else did either. Karen sat down next to Priya, clasped her arms around her and held her in a tight hug. She whispered over and over that it was going to be OK. Seeing close physical contact – proscribed within clinical areas during the pandemic – the observing nurse stood up as if to intervene. Dayan glared at her and she sat down again.

Hindsight is every doctor's friend. With an inflammatory process running rampant through her limbic system this combination of behavioural change, fluctuating conscious level and bizarre movements makes complete neurological sense. In fact, it is typical for this condition. But faced with a teenager acting strangely the doctors went down the psychiatric route and diagnosed an acute psychotic disorder. Recreational drugs are often suspected, but Priya had had none and all the tests were negative.

Priya was moved to a mental health unit, where she was given anti-psychotic medication to no avail. Twice over the next week she was observed to collapse and briefly lose consciousness: each time she was reassessed in the emergency department and then sent back again. Finally, Priya had what was clearly an epileptic seizure and was admitted to the hospital's medical wards. This in turn led to review by an experienced neurologist, who promptly diagnosed NMDA receptor encephalitis.

Such a misdiagnosis may seem shocking, but in fact the early stages of this condition are often dominated by mental health symptoms so this sequence of events is not unusual. NMDA encephalitis was only first described in 2007 and is often still overlooked. In my neurology clinic I once saw a woman, Sally, who had already spent six months on a psychiatric ward with a mysterious psychosis before the diagnosis was made.

For Priya, once this had happened things moved fast. She was transferred to our hospital, put into an induced coma and nursed on the Intensive Care Unit. Her blood was filtered and she was given a drug to switch off her antibody production entirely. Soon after she was moved her parents sat down for nearly an hour with the consultants and anaesthetists running the unit and discussed what they might expect. There was a sense of relief that Priya at least now had a diagnosis and was in the right place to be treated.

Priya's father remembers asking the ICU doctors how long she would take to get better. 'Will she have to stay in hospital for long?' he asked. 'Two or three weeks?'

He remembers a pause at this point, before the consultant replied, 'Patients with Priya's condition often stay on the Intensive Care Unit for several months. They are usually then in hospital for some months after that.'

Dayan and Karen had no response to this but a shocked silence.

Priya remained on the ICU for over three months, much of that time in an induced coma. Once the encephalitis had settled enough for her to be woken up, and her seizures were controlled, she was still a very long way from being herself. She continued initially to make odd movements, mainly gurning of her mouth, and was unable to swallow normally so would drool her saliva. Though she was now talking again, her memory was poor so she struggled to retain information. The childlike behaviour persisted to start with: as her mother put it, she woke up young. In this altered state, Priya was moved to our ward for rehabilitation.

*

The first actual human brain that I was allowed to handle belonged to Gladys. At least we called her Gladys, though none of us knew her real name. The anatomy department of my medical school had its own dissection room, and the introduction of a student to their cadaver was a rite of passage at the very start of a long training journey. For most this was also our first chance to find out whether we had the stomach for what was to come. Each body was shared between six students and would stay with us over two years of anatomy training, albeit in steadily smaller pieces.

The first session started with an hour spent crammed with sixty or so others into a Victorian lecture hall, steeply raked so that my knees pressed into the hard dark wood of the row in front. Once the anatomy professor had finished his talk – a detailed account of the muscles of the hand, delivered in a flurry of chalk dust – his assistant threw open the doors to the dissection room itself, with rather more drama than was strictly necessary. We shuffled through, in a nervous hubbub of exaggerated good cheer, and found ourselves in a large brightly lit space filled by two long rows of tables. The smell of formaldehyde was like a slap in the face.

We donned protective gowns and gathered around our assigned slabs, each adorned with a body-shaped lump wrapped in a thick plastic shroud. Pulling ours back revealed a smallish woman in her eighties, with not a stitch to cover her. Her remaining hair was shrunken down to thin wisps, and her skin was thickened and sallowed by the preserving process. On her slab she seemed small and alone, and the physical proximity of her death was palpable.

My first thought was that when this lady had presumably donated her body to medical science she may have imagined something rather different – a role in finding a cure for Parkinson's disease, perhaps. Instead she was to be reduced to her component parts by six teenagers. If she could see in from wherever she was then I could only hope she had a sense of humour. It was then that we decided that she must have a name, and Gladys seemed as good as any.

We were to seek out and dissect the Abductor Pollicis Brevis muscle, which is at the root of the thumb. I forget which of us made the first incision – a deep cut with a scalpel along half the length of her palm – but I remember how wrong it looked, an obscene bloodless chasm opening up in the intimate space of her hand. At least one student in the room fainted. The rest of us took deep breaths, swallowed hard and set to it.

The start of year two brought the prospect of the head and neck, between them complex enough to require a year of their own. Rather disconcertingly, all the heads had been removed from their trunks over the summer, so on arrival we were presented with one smaller polythene sack containing Gladys's head and a larger one for all of her other remains.

An old lady's head in a plastic bag. In almost any setting this is fundamentally very wrong, but by this point we were already fairly desensitised. To pick up a human body part and examine it as if it were an unusual bird's egg takes some getting used to. The first few times I could feel myself suppressing a physical sense of revulsion, having actively to instruct my hand not to let go of the severed arm. With time and practice the need to do this faded, as my mind slowly transferred the objects on the slab from the category of person to that of specimen. It was as if the connection in my brain linking the perception of a human form and my emotional reaction to it was being gradually weakened.

After months spent on the neck and the nerves of the face, the day finally came for the brain itself to be taken out. This was very much the business end of things as far as I was concerned, so when the top of the skull had been lifted off and the anatomy demonstrator opened out the fibrous layer of dura lying underneath it I felt my pulse begin to pick up. Peering down into the hole opening up beneath me, I felt the guilty thrill of an Egyptologist disturbing the Pharoah's tomb. It is hard to imagine a grosser violation of the repose and dignity of death – and yet here we were.

There inside sat the wrinkled form so familiar from textbooks. After gently reaching underneath it at front and back, and cutting away its underside from the nerves and blood vessels beneath, it was prised free and lifted out.

Now on the slab sat something resembling a small, wrinkly loaf of bread, but no ordinary loaf. This had a perfect symmetry and a folded complexity of form that was unfathomable. It looked like an object from another world. Seeing each gyrus looping around its neighbour, turning in folds like an endless ribbon – diving down from the surface into hidden depths before re-emerging and then round again, lobule on lobule, lobe on lobe – it was easy to believe that the secrets of an entire life lived within. It had been worth the months of leg muscles and kidneys to get to this.

No reverent hush descended. As I picked up the whole brain and held a gyrus between my fingers the clattering of scalpels continued, and the chatter and guffaws of fellow students echoed about the dissection room. And yet between my fingertips was a lifetime – love and laughter, niggles and pet peeves. A history both social and personal spanning a crazy century, from a childhood among streets smelling of horse manure all the way to Britpop.

It was hard to reconcile the yellow-grey sausage of each gyrus with the endless complexity of wiring that I knew lay within. It was in there somewhere, though, and for me that was enough.

*

When Priya arrived on our ward she had not stood up for over five months. I went to see her with our neuropsychologist Monica, and we found her in one of the side-rooms propped up in bed alongside a large furry bear. She looked as if she had gone twelve rounds with Tyson Fury. There was a scar on her breastbone where her thymus gland, an immune organ in the chest, had been removed as part of her treatment, bruises on her arms from endless blood tests and a tube from her stomach poking out from underneath her boyband T-shirt. Her signature pigtails were back in place but her face was slightly rounded from months of steroids. Leaning on her teddy and surrounded by get well cards, she seemed even younger than her years.

Priya looked downcast, but she brightened as we entered and greeted us with a cheery wave. I was briefly flattered by her enthusiasm but her eyes lit on Monica, whom she had met once before.

'I missed you!' she said, and squeezed Monica's hand. I introduced myself.

'Ooh, so you're the doctor. Are you going to make me better?'

'Well, I think you are the one who is going to do that, Priya – with a bit of help.'

I asked her a little about what she remembered of her illness. She was disinhibited and familiar in her manner, shooting conspiratorial grins at Monica from time to time. At first she was very attentive, asking quick-fire questions, but quite soon she began to become distracted.

'Would you like to meet Big Sam?' she asked, indicating her bear. Her intonation was more childish than teenaged. She asked Monica if she had a boyfriend and became rather sulky when we directed the conversation back to her. I asked how her mood had been – had she felt sad, or was she OK? She turned on a sixpence, looking suddenly horrified.

'Are you cross with me?'

She buried her face in Big Sam and sobbed. We reassured her that nobody was cross and within a minute she was giggly again. When we took our leave she told us that we had made her day, though I found this hard to believe.

Priya showed signs of several distinct but interacting difficulties. Neurologically her brain was still in the throes of a gradually resolving encephalitis and was functioning abnormally in a number of ways. If we could have taken a microscope to her brain we would have seen inflammatory cells clogging up the tissue in her hippocampus and disrupting the circuits which lay down new memories. We would likely have seen similar changes also in her amygdala and other regions of her limbic system, getting in the way of her emotional regulation and leading to the rapid fluctuations that were evident. The connections from her lower brain regions to her frontal lobes would be similarly affected, preventing her from planning her actions and engaging in strategic thinking.

Physically her body showed the effects of having been immobile for a long time and of the medical battering she had received. Psychologically she had been through what for anybody would be a terrifying experience, and as a teenager she was suffering the particular indignity of needing help going to the loo. It was our job to unpick the tangle of her many difficulties, make sense of them and set her on the path to recovery.

Rehabilitation is an ongoing process rather than a contained treatment and will continue long beyond the hospital admission. It is not confined to treatment sessions but rather is incorporated into everything the patient does and into every interaction they have. The brain performs so many different functions that when it goes wrong the range of therapeutic skills needed is wide, several professional disciplines each bringing their expertise to bear. Our patients will be assessed and treated by physiotherapists, occupational therapists, speech and language therapists, neuropsychologists, music therapists, dieticians, specialist nurses, social workers, rehabilitation assistants and a range of doctors. During a long hospital stay other figures may also become important members of the support network. The patient must be the main agent of change and should drive their own recovery, but of course when the brain is part of the illness then their capacity to do this may be altered.

The rehabilitation unit in its current multi-disciplinary form has come about gradually over many years and continues to evolve as patients' needs and our understanding shift. The idea that it is even desirable to restore damaged people to activity was not always a given. The ancient Greeks saw disability as a punishment from the gods for some misdeed, something to be hidden away. When the heroes of the epics were injured they usually either died on the spot or recovered quickly to win the day. They did not tend to linger in an altered state.

Hippocrates in Greece and the Roman Galen were certainly interested in the possibility of restoring lost function, but the idea largely fizzled out with the Dark Ages: it took the renewed interest in anatomy and mechanics that came with the Renaissance to rekindle the idea that you can promote recovery. Yet despite renewed interest the concept of rehabilitation remained a fairly amorphous affair. The convalescent homes which appeared in the countryside during the Victorian era, spurred on by urban disease and in particular by tuberculosis, offered decent sanitation, clean air and a nutritious diet. They provided an escape from those dark satanic mills but were not usually underpinned by any philosophy or method of recovery.

As so often, it was war that provided the impetus to progress. The industrial-scale maiming of an entire generation during the First World War created a subsequent need to get people mobile again and back into the workplace. This period also saw the first recognition of severe psychological injury resulting from trauma, and the (temporary) establishment of a dedicated rehabilitation facility at Craiglockhart in Edinburgh that treated, among others, the war poets Wilfred Owen and Siegfried Sassoon.

The concepts of physical therapy that were developed on the European battlefield were taken back to the US by the likes of John Stanley Coulter and applied to the civilian population. He was then joined by physician Frank Krusen in setting up some of the first rehabilitation units, and in pushing what was considered a fringe interest towards medical respectability. The entry of the US into the Second World War led to the establishment of large rehabilitation hospitals, and the polio epidemic of the 1950s further increased the need for a systematic approach to disability.

With growing recognition of this need, the nascent field of physiotherapy (or physiatry, or physical therapy – take your pick) aimed to restore more normal movement in the face of neurological impairment. This grew out of the late Victorian neurology concept of 'motor re-education' and was championed in London by a married couple, Jewish refugees from Berlin, Karel and Berta Bobath. Their approach took the principles of acquiring a new skill – motor learning – and applied them to the rehabilitation of movement. They emphasised the control of posture and the quality of the re-learned movements, avoiding the use of compensatory patterns and incorporating the new movements into everyday tasks. For some therapists the Bobath method is akin to a religion.

But there is clearly more to neuro-disability than difficulty controlling movement. The brain is our interface with the world, mediating the entire human experience. When it is damaged all sorts of changes may occur, and a focus on movement alone clearly misses the point. Since the late seventies we have increasingly understood that how we experience physical illness is inextricably linked with our psychological and social contexts, and that these aspects cannot meaningfully be separated – the 'biopsychosocial' model. Writing it down on the page now it seems blindingly obvious, which is a measure of how deeply embedded this approach has become in how we think about health and disease.

The key insight is to regard a person's level of functioning as a dynamic interaction between their physical health, environmental factors and personal factors. Your body's structures and functions (e.g. your brain controlling your legs) enable activities (e.g. walking), which in turn enable participation in society (e.g. going to the bingo). Conversely, when a health condition such as a stroke causes an impairment of your body's structures and functions (e.g. weakness down one side), this hampers your activities and participation (cannot walk to the bingo). Feeding into this chain of consequences are environmental factors (there is no ramp to get into the bingo hall) and personal factors (you cannot stand bingo anyway – who suggested it in the first place?).

Each new patient comes with a complex mish-mash of factors affecting their ability to function. The first thing the therapists will do is to make a list of their impairments, then of their activities and participation, and then of the environmental and personal factors which play a role. This provides a practical way of cutting through complexity but it also requires diagnostic skill and the ability to unpick a tangled knot.

A man recovering from a stroke may be unable to use a fork to feed himself (an activity) and so cannot join the other patients for lunch (participation). Why can he not use the fork? Has the stroke weakened the connection between the brain and his arm? Is there a disturbance of coordination, ataxia? Is there damage to the brain's store of motor programmes, apraxia? Maybe the stroke has affected sensation from that side and he cannot feel the fork properly? Does he have a problem with his eye movements, seeing two plates instead of one? Is there a gap in his visual field on one side, meaning that he cannot see the plate at all? Maybe his attention mechanisms are off kilter and he can see it but not notice it (hemispatial neglect)? Alternatively, he may have a medical cause for nausea and be off his food, or his low mood may have affected his appetite. Is the table too high to reach (environmental factors)? Maybe the ward forgot to order a Halal meal, or he just never liked beef stew anyway (personal factors). By dissecting out the impairments, you come to understand the obstacles preventing the activity and so can identify a potential route to restoring it.

On her first day with us Priya had a neurological examination and a long session with the therapy teams, who drew up a list of impairments: 1) weakness of all four limbs, due to muscle loss from lying flat; 2) reduced core stability; 3) shortening of the Achilles tendons (also from lying flat); 4) reduced balance; 5) reduced speed of information processing, naming, attention and recall; 6) reduced executive function (ability to initiate and organise activities); 7) reduced word fluency; 8) childlike behaviour with occasional temper tantrums; 9) some difficulties with continence; 10) intermittent anxiety.

As a result of these impairments her activities and participation were limited in a number of ways. She needed two people to help her wash or get dressed. She needed two people and some equipment to get her from bed to chair. She needed a wheelchair to get about and this needed to be pushed. She initially found it hard to maintain relationships with the staff as a result of her reduced emotional control. Communication with her family by phone was very difficult, as she found the process of having a conversation tiring and quite daunting. She would not even contemplate contacting her friends, as she was worried about how they would perceive her. The thought of going back to her sixth form college or considering a work role was so remote as to be off the radar.

Armed with this analysis, and with information from her family, the therapists and I sat down and drew out a diagram of Priya's difficulties and how these related to her ability to function, lists on a flipchart joined by arrows. This included her impairments but also factors intrinsic to Priya that were either predisposing to her difficulties or protective against them, as well as home and environmental factors that would play a role. Finally we tried to capture a sense of her values and what was important to her: music, ice-skating, her sister Geetha and socialising with her friends. This process served to make sure that everyone in her team had a similar understanding of what Priya was facing.

The next step was to make sure that Priya and her parents understood what was happening, and what we planned to do about it. Communication from the various medical teams had been very thorough from the time she was transferred to intensive care. Nonetheless, almost all of the focus to this point had been on the medical aspects of treating her encephalitis. Dayan and Karen had a good understanding of her condition, but they had not yet had a chance to understand how this linked to the complicated changes they could see in their daughter.

We met in a room off the main unit, a bright and airy space with light pouring in from a high window overlooking the square. Priya arrived in her wheelchair, and as Dayan pulled the door shut behind her the bustle of the ward receded. I asked her if she could remember what had happened and why she was in hospital. She looked uncertain.

'Is it . . . seizures?'

I nodded encouragement. 'Yes, you have had quite a few seizures, that's right. Luckily not for several weeks now though. But can you remember what it is that has caused them and made you unwell generally?'

Priya was struggling. She had been told this before, and had a simplified summary of her condition written down in a laminated booklet we had made for her, but she just could not access the information.

'It's called encephalitis, which means that your brain has been inflamed. Sometimes it can be caused by an infection, but in your case it was your own immune system taking a wrong turn. Instead of making antibodies to attack germs it made ones which interfered with your own brain and made it swell up.'

I pointed at an MRI scan which was up on the screen. The black and white image showed a slice through Priya's head as viewed from below, a high-quality picture almost like a photograph with clearly identifiable eyes, nose and ears. Having oriented Priya and her parents to these landmarks I indicated the squiggly mass in the middle as the brain, and as I scrolled up and down you could get a sense of its folds and its shape. On either side there were areas where the folds appeared different from their neighbours, thicker and with a hazy whiteness that gave an impression of swelling.

'These areas are the temporal lobes, and the parts in the middle are important for laying down memories and controlling your emotions,' I explained. 'Here you can see they look swollen, and when that happens people get pretty unwell. They often have epileptic seizures, are confused and forgetful, and become upset easily. Other brain areas are also affected, which can cause difficulty with movement and balance.'

Priya seemed to take this in.

'How long have I been in hospital?'

I told her it was just over six months and she raised her eyebrows wearily.

Karen and Dayan had some questions about medications, and what further treatment was needed for the encephalitis. As we talked I could see Priya mulling over what I had just been saying. She looked puzzled, as if she were groping for a thought or a question. I waited.

'But will I get better?' she asked finally.

'You are already so much better than a few weeks ago, and we expect you to keep improving,' I explained.

I told her that the most important thing she could do was to take part in the therapy we were offering her, but as I spoke her attention was beginning to wane and I realised I was losing her. Dayan took her back to her room but as he left he indicated that he had more to ask. When he returned, he sat next to Karen, took her hands in his and turned to me.

'Look, doc,' he said, 'we appreciate everything you are doing for Priya – everyone has been great – but we need a straight answer. Will she get back to normal? She is only a teenager, her whole life ahead of her. Will she fulfil her pot—'

His voice broke and his eyes filled. This was of course the million-dollar question, and one which at that point I could not fully answer. I explained that we had only just started intensive therapy and that it was hard to give an accurate answer just yet. When we had observed over a few weeks how Priya was responding we would have a better idea. I explained, with care, that after such a severe inflammation of the brain many people do show some long-term effects on their thinking skills, but that we see a wide range: in some it is quite marked while in others you would barely notice any change.

'Thanks for being honest, doc.'

But I could see from his flat expression that this was not what he had wanted to hear.

*

By now Priya had embarked on the therapy programme. Each week she was given a timetable of all her therapy sessions in advance. Monday to Friday she would take part in several sessions of forty-five minutes each day, including physiotherapy, occupational therapy and speech and language therapy. A neuropsychologist would work with her to assess her thinking skills and support her mood. Most of these would be one-to-one sessions, but for some she would take part in groups: brain injury group, breakfast group, exercise group, art group, pamper group. Every week the whole team would meet and we would discuss her progress, including medical, therapy and nursing aspects. The therapists would identify obstacles to her progress – pain, stiffness, mood fluctuations, continence issues – and we would troubleshoot to remove them.

This was all fairly overwhelming for Priya. Our endlessly patient charge nurse Dennis was a reassuring presence. With his kind face and soft lilting voice he had a calming effect on others amid the sometime chaos, and time seemed to slow down around him. He spent a lot of time reassuring Priya and explaining everything that was happening to her. As she was initially a little shy to come out of her room, Dennis gradually coaxed her out into the large day room where patients congregated and ate their lunch.

Priya sat at one of the tables and our rehab assistant Kevin set her up with something to do. In his strong north London accent he chatted away about Tottenham football club and showed her photos of Tina, his Staffordshire terrier. Watching from behind her desk was Nefertiti, our ultra-capable receptionist. Petite but all-powerful, and immaculate in a bright coloured headscarf, she made sure that everything was running as it should. Every so often she sharply upbraided Kevin and others for some minor misdemeanour, meting out good-humoured reproach with the ruthlessness of her namesake. Then the catering manager Vittorio emerged from the ward kitchen, gesticulating and volubly getting involved before being likewise cut down to size. This was typical ward cabaret and, despite herself, Priya had to laugh. Sitting in the day room's large space, bathed in sunlight and surrounded by activity, she began gradually to find the confidence to interact again with others. She rather took a shine to Christian, who was now taking all of his meals in the day room, and walking through I would often see them sharing a table in companionable silence over lunch.

The process of neurorehabilitation is structured around setting goals. Around two weeks into her admission the therapists produced a set of discharge goals for Priya, a list of what we thought she might be able to do by the time she left the unit –

an educated guess at this stage – and we shared these with her and her parents. This document covered all aspects of daily life and included a provisional discharge date set at four months from that point. She was also given a set of short-term goals, to be renewed every two weeks during her stay – stepping stones along the way. There is evidence that setting goals in this way increases participation and leads to better outcomes.

Priya helped us to set her discharge goals. She wanted to get home to see her friends and family, and in the meantime to explore ways to keep in contact with them. She wanted to walk on her own, go swimming and get back to running. She wanted to wash and dress herself, to go to the toilet on her own, and to style her hair. She wanted to get back to eating the things she liked, not to have a feeding tube in her stomach any more, and to make her own lunches and hot drinks.

She wanted to think clearly, and to manage her emotions. She wanted to understand her illness and how it had affected her body. She wanted to understand her medications and what they were for. She wanted her speech to be clearer, and to improve her writing. She wanted to think about what she might do in the future, maybe going back to college or doing an apprenticeship.

Priya's final goal was the most poignant.

'I want to like myself again.'

*

Historically, compensatory strategies have largely formed the mainstay of rehabilitation: using a frame to walk, for example, or learning to get dressed with one arm. However, it has gradually become apparent that in many patients you can change the impairment itself. By repetitive training, akin to learning a new dexterous skill, you can gradually re-train the patterns of movement until they more closely resemble the original. This change depends on repetitive practice in the hands of a skilled therapist and is driven by neuroplasticity, of which more later. This plasticity-driven training – or behavioural repair, as some prefer – is the engine of change in neurorehabilitation. Much of what we aim to do as a team is to create the ideal conditions for this process to occur, removing obstacles along the way. This requires multi-disciplinary working.

Around the time we were analysing Priya's difficulties, Christian's rehabilitation was underway, and multi-disciplinary problem solving was key to this getting going. When we first received him Christian was very weak on his left side and the therapists spent the early sessions working on transfers from his bed to a chair. With each attempt strong spasms would start up in his weak leg, knocking him off balance. We considered anti-spasmodic medication, but worried that this would make him drowsy. His spasms were exacerbated by an over-full bladder, by constipation (common after stroke) and by a sore area of skin on his bottom. This itself may in part have resulted from the spasms, pushing his rear end into the chair when he was seated.

By treating Christian's constipation, protecting his skin and ensuring that his bladder was not over-full, the spasms might well subside. If not, then a Botox injection to one or more of the leg muscles might do the trick. Another important factor for Christian was the anxiety he experienced around transfers, which would also set off the spasms. We asked our neuropsychologist to deliver joint sessions with the physios, applying distraction and other strategies to reduce his anxiety.

In order for this sort of multi-disciplinary unpicking of obstacles to work you need clear and effective communication between the several professionals involved, and you need the time and space to have that conversation. In a certain London neurorehabilitation unit the consultant used to conduct the ward round discussions standing by a grand piano, often for an hour or more, everyone remaining silent until spoken to. This form of old-school hierarchical working makes for a shorter ward round, but it does not allow complex problems to be unravelled in a way that works well for the patient – open discussion with a level hierarchy is the order of the day, and for good reason.

It was difficult at first to get going with Christian's therapy. Our therapists coaxed him out of bed each morning, but sometimes he would politely say, 'I can hear you, but I just want to sleep please!' We introduced medications to treat the pain in his left side, a common and often overlooked problem in stroke, and ramped up the doses until this settled.

The physiotherapists started taking Christian to the gym every day. They wheeled him down there in his tilting chair and then hoisted him out onto a plinth, a large padded rectangular slab used for physio. They propped him up on the plinth's edge but initially he could only manage to keep himself upright for fifteen seconds. He would lean back and to the left, so between two of them they rocked him forwards and backwards, shifting his weight gradually forward and getting him used to putting weight through his feet on the floor.

Christian would quickly get upset and anxious, asking for oxygen. The team persisted with reassurance and distraction until he could manage a session of nearly an hour. The physios set up a mirror in front of him so that he could begin to correct his own midline position when seated. They stretched out his tight hamstrings, helping him to straighten his left leg fully when trying to stand. They got him going on an enhanced exercise bike that provides just enough assistance to strengthen weakened limbs. They re-trained his movement into more effective patterns.

After six weeks of this, Christian no longer needed to be tilted and was able to sit next to his bed in a normal armchair. He was beginning to stand in physio sessions (supported, and with a left knee splint) and was trying transfers using a wooden sliding board as a kind of smooth bridge between bed and chair.

The occupational therapists began to get Christian involved with washing and dressing himself. These are complicated multi-stage activities engaging several cognitive processes, some of which had been affected by his stroke. To start with, the therapists would effectively move his limbs for him. From there they began using single-step written prompts – scrawled on the whiteboard – for each stage. 'Turn on tap. Put toothbrush onto basin. Squeeze toothpaste onto it.' He would get stuck on one stage when washing, repeatedly scrubbing one leg with the sponge. He had difficulty completing steps in the right order, forgetting to apply soap before scrubbing. He needed reminding to wash his left side and found it difficult to monitor what was going on around him, not noticing when the basin had filled up with water and began to overflow.

Initially Christian was dispirited by the difficulties he had performing what must have felt like simple tasks. Gradually though, with reassurance, repetition and small successes, he began to need less support and to feel more confident.

I came to visit one afternoon and found him looking dapper and groomed, the hospital gown replaced by his own T-shirt and a pair of tracksuit bottoms. I asked what he had been doing that morning and he broke out into a grin.

'Cooking curry!' he announced, his eyes twinkling.

To be honest I was a little sceptical but his report checked out. He had suggested this as a goal so his occupational therapist had helped him plan the recipe, make a list of ingredients and embark in his wheelchair to the local Waitrose. Back in our adapted kitchen they had given him a special spiked board, so that he could chop vegetables one-handed without them skidding about, and had helped keep him on track throughout the whole process. The therapists told me that he had lit up, humming and singing while he cooked. I missed out on the resulting curry, but then the consultant always does.

Such minor victories go a long way, and Christian's morale turned a corner post-curry. Week by week his life was becoming more bearable, the grinding rhythm of his daily routine increasingly studded by small victories. The prospect of returning to his flat began to seem less of a pipe dream and, after three months of intensive work, we got him home. He was supported initially with four daily visits from a carer to help with getting washed and dressed but he could take part in these tasks. Once he was up and dressed he could get on with his day.

I visited Christian and Julie at their home a few months later. Their flat sat within an Edwardian redbrick mansion block tucked into a busy industrial area of London. The block was surrounded at front and side by a secluded communal garden, a line of plane trees screening out the city beyond. As I stepped into the relative calm of their shade my mind cast back to the distressed figure I had first met dangling in a hoist from the ceiling, robbed of his dignity by pain, helplessness and the need for a pad change.

Julie buzzed me into the building then met me at the door to their flat. Gone was the tracksuit. She wore a plain but elegant shift, covered from the waist with a pinny, and judging from the sweet smell in the hall she had been baking. She gave me a generous hug and ushered me through into their kitchen-sitting room, where I found Christian sitting at the table with a large grin on his face. He had his weaker left hand up on the tabletop with the fingers stretched out – as our therapists had taught him – and with his right hand had been helping Julie prepare some sort of sweet scone.

We drank tea, ate a little and chatted. I complimented them on the scones. Christian gave me a conspiratorial smile and indicated Julie.

'Yes, prison food. She is the warden!'

He laughed and his eyes lit up the kitchen. For the first time since we met I could picture him as he would have been previously, smartly dressed in a tuxedo and energetically mixing a Manhattan. The two of them demonstrated how they could now get him on and off the sofa using a small wooden sliding board. Each day he stood up with some support for about twenty minutes at a time. The local borough's physio had been working some more with him, and he had begun to take a few steps. His left arm remained weak but he had learned how to use it a little, for example holding a shower gel bottle while washing himself.

I asked how much they were able to get out of the flat. Julie was confident enough to take Christian outside in his wheelchair to the communal garden each morning. They could sit outside with a cup of tea, soak up the sounds of the street and chat to neighbours. They could also visit the local shops and go to church on Sunday.

I took my leave, and Julie walked me to the door. Before she closed it behind me she paused in the doorway.

'I did get him back.'

As I made my way back down to the courtyard I pondered how their life had changed. Christian was still significantly disabled to be sure, but he had a quality of life and a level of dignity that by any standard was decent.

I did the sums: the cost to the taxpayer of Christian's neuro-rehabilitation stay would have been around £40,000. This sounds like a lot of money, but during this admission the estimated cost of his care needs fell by £2,640 per week. In other words, the cost of his rehabilitation to the national purse would have been offset within less than four months of his going home, and would potentially go on to save tens or hundreds of thousands in the longer term. Most importantly, Christian got to go home with Julie.

*

For Priya, meanwhile, the obstacles to achieving her goals were very different. Her progress on the physical front was relatively quick. The physios identified the aspects that were holding her back and worked these hard. After around six weeks of intensive therapy she had progressed from needing a sliding board for her transfers to walking short distances with a Zimmer frame. Priya had the advantage that the pathways from her brain to her limbs were essentially intact, unlike Christian for example, but for her the motor system was not the main issue. In fact, the more alert and mobile she became the more the changes in her thinking became apparent.

Monica came to see her for a neuropsychology session early on and found her standing up in front of her wheelchair. Priya's Zimmer frame was a couple of yards away out of reach and the wheelchair footplates were sticking out in front of her legs, about to trip her up if she moved forward. Monica asked her if the physios had yet given her the all-clear to walk on her own. Priya burst into tears.

'I don't know, but I need the toilet and I've had enough!'

Monica put an arm around her, allowed her to calm down, and asked one of the nurses to help get her to the loo.

Priya called these her crying fits, and she had a few each day to start with. For a young person stuck in hospital and needing help with toileting this seemed to me an entirely reasonable reaction. But once Monica got her settled for her psychology session it became clear that on this day there was more to it than general frustration. She had finally retrieved her phone from her parents, anxious to look on social media and see what her friends had been up to, but she could not remember the code. When Monica helped her to find her Instagram account on a desktop PC she could not get into that either and had trouble navigating her way about the site. When Monica then supported her in sending an old-fashioned email to a friend she became nervous, and struggled to put a sentence together. This led her to become upset again.

Dayan and Karen were often on the ward and were unfailingly

supportive, but we could see them beginning to realise that despite the physical gains there was still a long way to go. The society that we have created for ourselves places much emphasis on our analytical and social thinking skills and is relatively unforgiving when they falter. It was clear that helping Priya with this was going to be central to her recovery. As so often when unpicking our patients' difficulties, we would have to open that great black box: cognition.

CHAPTER THREE

GRIT IN THE COGS

When I started my medical training I was convinced that as a qualified doctor I would be spending a lot of time performing CPR. When confronted with a cardiac arrest my 'training would kick in', and I would slip automatically into a sequence of heroic actions that would bring the patient back from the brink. From what I knew about it then, you pumped your arms up and down on the chest for a while, shouted 'Clear!', delivered a few electric shocks and injected intravenous adrenaline. The patient would usually then take a deep breath, open their eyes and sit up. There would follow a scene of tearful gratitude.

This airbrushed impression came largely from a late 1990s TV diet, my Friday nights spent watching *ER* (after *Friends* and *Frasier* – obviously I would then go out and have an amazing social life). Thinking about it now, it is worrying just how much of my general medical knowledge that show provided. While I did indeed perform plenty of CPR as a junior doctor the reality was rather different. It somehow lacked the glamour of the Chicago emergency room, and not just because I was doing much of it in Luton.

The patient's body does not jump off the bed with each shock, but just sits there. Nurse Hathaway is nowhere to be seen. More importantly, what you miss on the TV shows is the state the patient is in after their brain has been starved of oxygen for several minutes.

As a houseman in a far-flung hospital I was paged one night from the respiratory ward. My 'bleep' was on the bedside table in my box-like on-call room, and it sprang harshly to life next to my ear. I surfaced from a fitful and all-too-brief sleep and checked my watch. It was 2.30 a.m. I fumbled for the bedside phone and dialled the number on the pager. It was Henry, one of the staff nurses on the night shift.

'Good morning, doctor, sorry for disturbing you.'

'That's OK, Henry, what's up?'

In calm and measured tones, Henry informed me that there was a problem with Mr Morris in bed 17.

'What sort of problem?'

'I cannot detect his blood pressure.'

Henry's voice conveyed all the urgency of the midnight shipping forecast. I sat up and swung my legs over the edge of the bed, reaching for my white coat on the foam chair. I was now fully awake.

'Well, is he breathing?'

'Hold on, doctor.' There was a clunk as Henry put the receiver onto the desk, and echoing footsteps as he went to check and then came back again. 'No.'

'Does he have a pulse?'

'Hold on.' Another clunk and what sounded like a leisurely stroll to investigate. 'No, there is no pulse.'

'Well, how long has he been like that for?'

'I am not sure.'

'Henry, what you are telling me is that Mr Morris is dead. Is he meant to be for resuscitation?'

'Let me check.' Another long pause. 'No, he is not for resuscitation.'

I took a deep breath and tucked my feet back under the blanket.

'That's lucky. OK, Henry, I'll come down to certify the death in a few minutes.'

Mr Morris was quite rightly not for resuscitation, having advanced emphysema that would have made the unpleasant process entirely futile. It is fair to say that Henry was not that ward's star nurse, and these days proceedings would, I hope, have been rather slicker. But I had not appreciated as a student how poor the odds are for those who receive CPR. Even now, if your heart stops while you are in a hospital, and the resuscitation team come running, your chances of leaving hospital alive are around one in five. If you are not in a hospital at the time then this goes down to less than one in ten. For every minute of delay in starting CPR the odds of survival drop by 10 per cent.

The outcome after CPR depends to a degree on the quality of the technique and on how long it takes to get the heart working again. The brain is very demanding, chomping its way through energy like an overheating laptop just to keep all the neurons ticking over. In lightbulb terms it uses around 20 watts at rest: about a fifth of the body's overall energy demands from less than 2 per cent of its mass. Human brains are more than three times as demanding as those of other primates. This sounds like a positive, and it is – until the supply is interrupted.

To meet this demand the profligate brain tissue needs its blood supply to be of decent pressure, and to contain plenty of glucose and oxygen. If any of these are lacking then the metabolic demand soon outstrips supply. About five minutes after a cardiac arrest the brain tissue starts to accumulate permanent damage, and the longer the interruption the more extensive this is.

Once a blood pressure is restored further problems may yet develop. The automatic regulation of blood vessels is initially out of whack: the arteries dilate, allowing a surge of blood into the capillaries. This is akin to the red flaring-up of skin which you sometimes see after taking a tourniquet off your arm. In the brain this influx of blood increases the back pressure inside the skull, paradoxically reducing the perfusion pressure. This and a build-up of toxic metabolites in the tissues cause a secondary injury to the affected areas.

Medical treatment in this situation is focused on optimising conditions to minimise this secondary injury. Actively cooling the brain slows metabolism and may reduce this damage. Hippocrates seemed to know this and is said to have packed wounded soldiers into ice. It has also long been observed that drowning victims do better than expected if they are also hypothermic. Advocates of therapeutic hypothermia point to improved long-term outcomes in some trials, though its use is far from universal.

Although the whole brain is affected, the grey matter – where the neurons' demanding cell bodies are – is particularly vulnerable. The result is a characteristic pattern of damage which you can see on an MRI scan, affecting in particular the cerebral cortex around the brain's edge, the deep nuclei at its centre and the hippocampi.

Without a functioning hippocampus you could not lay down or retrieve any short-term memories. Without a functioning cerebral cortex you would have no awareness. Often after such a brain injury patients will therefore enter a period of coma, and whether they will emerge into wakefulness or remain in a state of low awareness is surprisingly hard to predict. Hypoxic brain injury is becoming increasingly common as more people survive cardiac arrest, but most do not fare well. Many never leave hospital. In those who wake up we may see a range of difficulties depending upon the extent and location of the damage. These may include physical impairments but the most striking changes are usually in thinking skills.

The role of neuroplasticity in recovery has been studied mainly in relation to movement, but the same principles likely apply equally to the rehabilitation of cognition. Patients rely heavily on their cognitive faculties to implement what they learn in therapy, so assessing these is an important part of the rehabilitation process.

*

Anton was in his late twenties when he came to us. He was a junior radiographer, a hard-working man from a conservative eastern European country who had arrived in the UK as a teenager. Anton liked to party. On a big night out he took something he shouldn't and collapsed in a club. He was in cardiac arrest so his horrified friends started CPR and called an ambulance: in total there was a ten-minute 'downtime' before the paramedics got his heart restarted.

Anton spent a month on the Intensive Care Unit in an induced coma, beset by epileptic seizures and with a breathing tube in his trachea, which was then converted to a tracheostomy. Once all sedation was stopped he was very slow to wake up.

I saw him with the therapy team soon after this. He had a slight frame, delicate features and cheekbones that you could shave with. He was propped up in the bed, but his eyes were closed, his head lolling to one side and his arms inert beside him. We greeted him but with no response, so I gently pressed one of his arms. Very slowly his eyes opened and he looked up, but he seemed to have difficulty making me out and was too sleepy to talk.

Around a month later the tracheostomy was out and he had woken up enough to come onto our unit. He was in the bay opposite the nurses' station – the builders were still working on the Bay 4 refurb – and I went to see him with our charge nurse Dennis. Anton was more upright in bed than previously, was more awake and could slowly move his arms. I asked how he was feeling. There was a long wait while he thought about this. When it came his voice was slow, and his syllables disjointed.

'Everything . . . looks very . . . strange.'

I waited.

'I cannot see you . . . clearly, and things are . . . moving around.'

As Anton's alertness improved so the effects of his hypoxic brain injury became more apparent. He had weakness on both sides of his body. There was stiffness in his limbs due to spasticity. The muscles and tendons in his shoulders and elbows had also tightened up and shortened from immobility. He could move his limbs but had poor coordination, so his movements were jerky and inaccurate. There was a partial loss of sensation which made accurate movements even harder.

As a result of these physical limitations Anton was entirely dependent: he needed help to sit up and hoisting to get out of bed. He was fed through a tube in his stomach. But for all this his most striking impairments had nothing to do with movement: Anton could hardly see and his thought processes were obviously clouded. Immobile, foggy-headed and partially blind – a frightening combination.

Anton's visual symptoms needed to be teased apart carefully. He could read a letter or word that was right at the centre of his visual field but only if it was quite large. He struggled to detect objects in his peripheral vision or even slightly away from the centre, especially to the left, but could easily distinguish different colours. He could detect visual targets more reliably if they were moving than if they were still (like a Tyrannosaurus rex, if *Jurassic Park* is to be believed). Anton had great difficulty separating out a visual scene into its components – confronted with a busy environment, he just could not distinguish the elements of what he was seeing. If you asked him to locate the water jug on his tray he would struggle, so the prospect of a busy street scene was overwhelming. While we were with him an enormous dog was brought into the bay – truly huge, like a Shetland pony – and he did not notice it.

As if this were not enough Anton was also plagued initially by a constant stream of visual hallucinations. He described seeing circles like Catherine wheels spinning about to either side of him. In the dark of the evenings he would see faceless mannequins sitting in the bay, seeming to peer at him from all sides. These figures would not move, and luckily he did not find them threatening, but they were an almost constant presence.

When talking to Anton he struggled to focus his attention, appeared forgetful and was very slow in his responses. To start with he would mix up the time of day, though this improved. He would get stuck on a topic and have difficulty switching to another. After a few minutes of speaking he would be exhausted.

Our cognitive functions are arranged in a modular fashion, with a number of distinct and specialised brain networks performing specific tasks. The nature of the difficulties a patient experiences depends on the anatomy of the damage. We could see patchy areas of abnormal brain on Anton's scan, but in order to help him it was necessary to understand which aspects were working well and which were not. Neurologists who work in dementia talk about 'taking a walk around the brain'. This means going through a series of questions with the patient, each depending upon a different brain region, until you have some idea where the problems lie.

A full cognitive assessment is most accurately done by a neuropsychologist and takes a while, but a shorter version done at the bedside can give you much of the information you need. Most neurologists who trained in London have a copy of the 'little green book', a laminated series of twenty or so tasks. This was developed by the pioneering neuropsychologist Elizabeth Warrington, a presence at Queen Square since the 1950s, and was designed to fit into a side pocket of the now extinct white coat.

By leading somebody through the book's questions you get a virtual tour of the brain's cognitive skills. Can they recognise famous faces (bottom of the temporal lobe)? Can they remember faces after an interval (inner right temporal lobe)? Can they remember a sequence of digits (part of the frontal lobe), or recall them backwards (another part of the frontal lobe)? Can they name some uncommon objects from drawings (bottom of left frontal lobe)? Can they identify a capital letter that has been broken down into fragments (connection between occipital lobes and right parietal lobe)? And so on.

Anton showed very slow information processing, likely from damage to the fast white matter connections linking remote brain regions. He showed a number of traits suggestive of frontal lobe damage: poor working memory (the mental buffer, used when you remember a phone number before writing it down), difficulty with abstract reasoning, such as interpreting proverbs non-literally, and distractibility. His actual memory seemed to be fine, but his ability to use it was compromised by trouble maintaining attention.

How can you fix these cognitive difficulties? Well, you cannot fix them directly, but by understanding them you can challenge them in a functional context – something meaningful like brushing your teeth or making a cup of tea – and devise strategies that will overcome them (I say 'you' can do this but I really mean occupational therapists). With constant practice the functions themselves may also improve. In Anton's case his visual difficulties added a further layer of complexity.

The therapists would break each task down into a sequence of steps – take the lid off the toothpaste, pick it up, use the other hand to keep the toothbrush steady, squeeze on the toothpaste, put it down, and then bring hand to mouth and get brushing. They would set everything up such that Anton could identify objects by touch, and would then use 'backward chaining' to help him re-learn the skill. This means starting off by doing everything for him except for the last step, in this case the actual brushing.

Once he had mastered that they would add in the previous step – squeezing on the toothpaste – and do everything for him to that point. They would then gradually work their way backwards along the sequence until he could do it from scratch.

The therapists used a similar approach for getting dressed and took advantage of Anton's visual strengths by colour coding his clothes drawer. He was quite particular about his clothing and appearance. Passing his bay in the morning I would sometimes see him sitting on the edge of his bed working slowly through his morning routine, his gaunt frame almost translucent against the light beyond. With one arm on the bed for support he would lean slowly forward and reach a jerky arm into his drawer to select a T-shirt. It was painstaking work but he seemed in no hurry.

*

A living brain looks quite different from a dead one. Salmon-coloured and spongy in substance, studded with small bright red vessels, it throbs gently in time with each heartbeat. Some years after the dissection room I found myself in an operating theatre, fully scrubbed in surgical gown and mask, and standing stock still while holding a suction catheter against a hole in a man's skull. My job was to suck up any blood that appeared as the operation progressed. As a relatively new junior doctor I was having a brief flirtation with neurosurgery as a career choice, so I spent six months as the skivvy of the team to get a feel for it. I realised fairly quickly that it was not for me. There were many reasons for this, but if you have ever seen me trying to carve a chicken then you would understand why a different direction was in everybody's interest.

I was excited to start the new post, but soon discovered that my work was in fact based entirely on the ward and had little or nothing to do with operating. As one of three Senior House Officers on the team (SHOs: the name is deceptive – we were the lowest of the low), my primary role was to make sure that patients were prepped and ready for surgery. We were also to gather up their brain scans for the operation and then look after their medical needs once they were back on the wards. As far as the consultants were concerned we were seen and not heard.

Finding CT scans was a lot harder than it sounds. These were actual physical scans, large acetates in square paper packets, and although in theory you could track their whereabouts on a computer system I quickly discovered that they could be almost anywhere in the hospital. This meant that the most important person for me to keep sweet was the lady who checked the scans in and out of radiology in the basement. Hours of my life were spent flicking through large metal trolleys full of scans, desperately searching for the all-important packet without which no operation could go ahead. My friend Ben failed to locate a scan in time for a planned tumour resection: the consultant told him to fuck off out of theatre.

After months of donkey work an opportunity to try my hand at operating came by chance one morning when one of the neurosurgical registrars – the actual surgical trainees – turned up uncharacteristically late. Each morning started at seven forty-five with a meeting around an X-ray viewing box. The registrar who had been on call overnight would put up the scans from new admissions, and the consultant would pick out one of us SHOs and ask what we saw. This was our chance to show that we could at least read a brain scan.

On this morning he turned to me. The consultant – tall, lean and immaculate in a three-piece grey suit – told me that the scan belonged to a sixty-two-year-old man who had fallen over in the street, possibly under the influence. He had struck his head and was found in a drowsy state. What could I see? There was a bright area on the scan, beneath the skull but overlying the brain's left hemisphere, which looked like an acute subdural haematoma resulting from trauma. This was a few centimetres across and was pushing the brain over towards the other side, so-called midline shift. The brain tissue itself underneath the clot also had flecks of blood and patchy dark areas within it, which suggested bruising and damage within the left frontal and temporal lobes. I said so, and to my relief the dapper consultant nodded approvingly.

At this point, around five minutes into our meeting, the operating registrar for that day appeared. She was bleary-eyed, dishevelled and looked like she had slept in her clothes. The consultant told her icily that turning up late was unacceptable: she should go away and come back when she was cleaned up. If she could not be bothered to show up on time then he would get one of the SHOs (me) to stand in for her in theatre. In fact, as I later found out, the registrar was diabetic and had suffered a nasty hypoglycaemic attack that morning.

So, drafted into some actual brain surgery on the back of the registrar's humiliation, I held onto my suction catheter and tried not to move a muscle. The consultant had made a largeish hole in the patient's skull using a hydraulic circular saw, and now he stood across from me looking down into it. We could see that the dura mater – the thick white fibrous layer that overlies the brain's surface – was bulging worryingly from within. He made an incision in it and as soon as he did so fresh blood oozed out, an ugly red stain creeping across the clean white membrane like paint across a canvas. I got my suction catheter in and off we went, the boss opening the dura out further and me removing the partly clotted blood. After a while all the blood was gone and the surface of the underlying brain peeped into view. Rather than the usual smooth loops of gyri the brain's appearance was speckled and bruised, like a piece of chicken to which somebody had taken a mallet. The blood clot now gone, the consultant stitched up the dura (I was allowed to cut the stitches), replaced the skull's bone flap and finally sewed the scalp back into place. Job done.

Back on the ward I discovered from the man's sister that his name was Paul and he was a sometime bricklayer. He had struggled with life generally for a few years and had been tipsy when he fell in the street. As the anaesthetic wore off Paul gradually surfaced, opening his eyes only briefly but long enough for me to do a quick assessment. He made eye contact and tried to speak but was unable to get any words out. He lifted up his left arm when I encouraged him, but his right arm was a dead weight. This was all in keeping with an injury to the left cerebral hemisphere.

Over the next few weeks I stopped in on Paul from time to time during my on-calls. These shifts were long and punishing, stretching continuously every fourth weekend from Saturday morning through to Monday evening. Over these fifty-six hours I would not leave the hospital but wandered back and forth between the ward, the canteen and the on-call room (and, rarely, the operating theatre), a disembodied zombie drifting about the scuffed linoleum corridors in an increasingly shabby white coat. In this particular hospital some genius had put the on-call rooms around the back of the operating theatres and on the same cold air ventilation system. This meant that the bed on which I snatched the odd spell of sleep was in a room which was literally refrigerated.

After a few weeks of trekking the long corridors between the ward and my ice box I discovered a secret rubbish lift that linked the back of the theatres with a corridor just next to the neurosurgery ward. If I crouched down and held my nose then I could be on the ward and rubbing my eyes within two minutes of my bleep going off.

We were Paul's local hospital, which meant that he was stuck on our ward until somewhere could be found for him to go. He had been living in a shared private rental, but there was no prospect of his managing there in his current state. He was at least alive thanks to the surgery but he was pretty disabled, unable to speak or to sit up in bed without support.

Each morning we would do a quick pre-theatre ward round with the registrars, but the focus was on the patients who were due for surgery or had just been operated on. Pushing the notes trolley past Paul's bed we would barely break step, and in the medical notes we would scrawl 'Impression: status quo, Plan: await placement.'

After a couple of weeks of this I began to wonder how Paul was ever supposed to improve. He was in a side-room, so was cut off from the chatter of the open ward. For almost all of his time in that room he lay in bed staring at a blank wall and he developed an increasing flatness in his eyes as his spirits gradually sagged. I could see that he was getting a little movement back in his right arm, but nobody was working with him to develop it. The only physios on the ward were busy treating chest infections, and in those days there was little or no structured therapy input to promote recovery. His quality of life in that side-room was pretty grim and there seemed no prospect of improving it.

I asked the nurses to sit him out in a chair for an hour or two in the day, and he seemed to perk up a little when he was more vertical than horizontal. He was still not speaking, but I discovered that if you jotted a few words down for him to choose from then he could usually point to one in order to answer a simple question. Pain? Yes/No. Where? Draw a picture of a stick man and ask him to point. He insistently indicated a plastic bag in the corner of the room, and in it I found a postcard of an idyllic seaside town – fishing boats bobbing in a blue bay in front of a row of pretty houses. It said 'Galway' at the bottom, and having established that this was his home town I propped it up on the corner of his window where he could see it. Paul responded with a thumbs-up and a crinkly, lop-sided smile.

I had worked out a reasonable means of communication, but at this point I was making it up as I went along: there was no speech therapist on hand to show me how to communicate properly with an aphasic patient. I thought about finding a therapist on another ward and persuading them to come and see him. Before I could do this, though, I turned up one morning to find a pre-surgical patient in his place: Paul had been discharged to a nursing home. I found the postcard on the floor in a dusty corner of the room.

*

As Anton began to settle in, Priya was still with us, working on her goals. She had a very different cognitive profile to Anton's. She was not particularly slow, and her early memory difficulties had largely resolved, but some frontal lobe functions were lagging behind. She was still quite disinhibited, struggled with abstract reasoning and was inflexible, finding it hard to switch between activities. The neuropsychologist Monica helped her write out a storyline of her illness, and gradually they built this up into a scrapbook. Monica and our speech therapist videoed Priya in conversation and played this back to her, allowing her to observe the changes in her communication and work on them. Priya could see from the video that she often wandered off topic, was distracted by something or became quickly upset. By completing such exercises together, they helped to build up Priya's confidence in how she communicated with others.

Priya worried that her friends might be moving on with their lives without her, but at the same time the prospect of speaking to them on the phone scared her: might she become overwhelmed or embarrass herself? With Monica she developed a series of written scripts for such situations, so that she would feel confident in dealing with them. 'Because of my encephalitis I might say goodbye quickly or get angry more quickly', or 'My encephalitis can make me a bit inappropriate, but it's nothing against you. You can tell me.'

As weeks turned into months, Priya kept drilling her cognition with Monica, alongside all the physical and functional work, and she began to feel more confident in speaking to people. Halfway through her admission Priya had to spend three days back on the ICU, for a planned procedure to filter out any remaining antibodies. Walking slowly in with her frame she was astonished when the charge nurse Jenny exclaimed 'Hello, stranger!' and clasped her in a hug. In fact all the staff there recognised her and greeted her like an old friend: and yet she had little or no memory of being there. She had, after all, been semi-comatose at the time.

As we gradually expanded Priya's horizons – home visits, trips into the local area – her remaining cognitive difficulties became more apparent. It seemed they were going to be slower to change, so we had to start considering how she might mitigate them when she moved on from the relative protection of our hospital to the world beyond.

*

When we learn and practise a new skill – or re-learn an old one – we must necessarily alter how we perform it. Making a movement in an identical way each time will not achieve anything: we must vary it slightly, detect when a change results in an improvement and then reinforce that change. So even if the goal is a more accurate and stable action, in order to reach that point we must paradoxically introduce a degree of variability and instability early on, casting about as a way of discovering how to get there. In other words, to improve we must experiment.

When I was around five years old I had a friend called Sophie who lived in the same street and we would play together at weekends. She had long wavy brown hair, nice teeth and knew a lot of secrets. We would sit together beneath the kitchen table and make up games, or watch *Doctor Who* nervously from behind the sofa. I rather wanted to impress her, and one day I told her proudly that when I grew up I was going to be an inventor. To me this seemed impossibly glamorous, an extension of the Heath Robinson posters on my bedroom wall. In my mind I pictured pulleys, levers and possibly trap doors. But Sophie shook her head. 'Oh no,' she said confidently, 'inventors are only paid one pound per week.' So that was that.

Though my inventing plans were scotched I longed to play around with things and to experiment. I picked this up, I think, at home, where experimentation was rife. While Sophie and I were scheming under the kitchen table my father was upstairs writing music in his loft workroom, kneeling on the floor with dozens of pieces of paper arranged around him. I would sometimes sit underneath his grand piano and watch him lost in thought, amid the smell of paper, rubbers and India ink. With his seventies-length dark hair and French nose, he was lost in a world of sound. As a young composer he had become fascinated by applying mathematical structures to creating sounds, modes of notes and shapes of phrases determined by patterns within intricate number grids. As he moved the scraps of paper about he was creating in his head a soundscape to describe the creation myth – the first dawning of light in the universe. Having completed this he went on to incorporate polyphonic west African structures into his composition (which involved spending months walking through rural Gambia with a tape recorder), studying with Olivier Messiaen in Paris and a long detour into electronic music (picture our loft filled with wires, gizmos and early synthesisers).

This sort of restless creativity is exhilarating if a little exhausting. But for me it exemplifies how we learn and grow. When trying to improve in an activity we must vary how we do it, exploring the 'performance space' and then locking in the changes when a new attempt is more successful – a kind of learning by natural selection. I saw this in my father's writing process, and I see it in patients recovering.

Learning a golf shot is an example of the sort of task to which this might apply: small, possibly random, changes in how the club is swung allow the learner to explore what works better and what does not. Too much variability and you would be unable to stabilise in the ideal state, but too little and you would not stray far enough to find it – in between there is presumably a sweet spot. Years later, with colleagues, I incorporated this concept into a mathematical model of this form of learning, and of how brain stimulation might enhance it, though we were hardly the first to use the idea.

For me such innovation and reinvention are essential ingredients of a certain kind of progress, whether in arts, science or even rehabilitation. From Newton to Bowie, having the space and the inclination to try things out have been key to making great things happen. This is effectively play, crucial in artistic endeavour and child development but also, I think, when recovering from brain injury. It is hard in a ward setting to create the right conditions for this play to take place, but this is what we try to achieve for our patients.

*

If our thinking skills are disrupted then often our behaviour will also change. In Anton we saw an exaggerated sloth of response, as if his cogs were grinding their way through treacle, while in Priya we saw a childlike playfulness and sometimes petulance. Patients in whom memory is significantly disrupted will often show frank confusion. In some this will lead in turn to agitation or even aggression, which may be hard to manage. In a rehab context there is an inherent contradiction: too little stimulation will hinder neuroplasticity and recovery but too much will exacerbate restless behaviour. You need staff who are experienced in behavioural management, neuropsychology input, ideally also mental health nurses, and certainly a psychiatrist. It is helpful to have access to a low-stimulation environment – a quiet bay away from the hurly-burly – and some units are set up exclusively for this purpose. The involvement of security guards is usually a sign that things have not gone according to plan.

Sometimes, though, when patients cross a behavioural line it is enough to clarify boundaries. Ray was a thickset man in his sixties with an unruly mass of ginger curls. He had been in prison for most of his adult life for killing a man in a bar fight in his reckless twenties, but he had a large stroke soon after being released. Although he engaged well in therapy he also began to play up with the staff. He refused personal care from certain nurses and began to make suggestive comments to female therapists. His physiotherapist had fitted a splint to his left ankle. As she knelt before him to adjust it Ray leaned forward and leered at her with what he probably thought was cheeky banter but in fact came across as classic dirty old man.

'You can help me out with something else while you're down there, love!'

I went to speak to Ray accompanied by our matron, a large bald German man with a basso profundo voice. We took him to an interview room and gave him a written warning about his behaviour, including consequences if he were to continue. We asked him to sign a behavioural contract if he wanted to remain with us. I was not holding out much hope for this approach but to my surprise it had a miraculous effect. We would still get the chat and jokes but he became helpful and compliant, going out of his way to help staff and the other patients. I realised that after years in prison Ray saw our ward as a similar environment: I was the governor, and the nurses were the screws. He called me Basil Fawlty, and one of the therapists was Manuel. We would joke with him about his 'release' date, and when he was eventually discharged he was genuinely missed.

A lack of behaviour can be as disabling as an excess. Tania was in her fifties and had a bleed around the brain that damaged her orbitofrontal cortex, which is important in initiation – your get-up-and-go. According to a standard neurological examination Tania was completely intact. She had full power in her limbs, normal coordination and sensation. You could engage her in conversation, and if asked to do so she could get up and walk. Sitting drinking tea in our day room – a quiet demeanour, short grey perm and glasses – she might have been running the cake stall at a village fete. And yet she was entirely dependent on care for everything. Her Barthel score (a measure of independence) was zero out of twenty.

Tania had no initiation at all and needed prompting to do even basic tasks. If you put a plate of food in front of her she would sit and look at it. If she needed the loo she would not call for help. This 'abulia' is very disabling and presents a problem for rehabilitation. We gave her a medication to stimulate the dopamine receptors in her frontal lobes and, with time and intensive therapy, she began to do things for herself.

People with cognitive change after brain injury are often vulnerable to the actions of others or themselves. Protecting a patient who is cognitively impaired can be clear-cut, for example if a visitor takes their bank card and asks them for their PIN number or asks them to sign legal documents on the ward (this happens more often than you might think). But it is sometimes less straightforward.

A senior barrister called Malcolm who had suffered a large right-sided stroke started working from his laptop on the ward, giving legal advice to clients. Malcolm had trouble sequencing the steps involved in making a cup of tea but was reviewing legal briefs. His judgement was certainly altered, so should we advise him not to give advice that might cause him reputational damage or even leave him liable? Would we be liable ourselves if we did not actually stop him?

Larry was a man in his fifties who survived a cardiac arrest but sustained a hypoxic brain injury in the process. He was slow to change and remained extremely cognitively impaired after three months. Larry's girlfriend Sherry introduced herself as his fiancée and we had no reason to doubt this, but alarm bells rang when she started making arrangements to marry him in the hospital chapel. We explained that as Larry currently did not know where he was he was hardly in a position to make a lifelong commitment. We thought the matter settled until Sherry was found sneaking onto the ward the following week with a chaplain discreetly in tow. Fortunately a therapist intervened.

*

Anton's therapy was progressing. Alongside the nuts and bolts of washing and dressing the physiotherapists got to work on his mobility, stretching out the muscles, building strength in the limbs and trunk and re-training common movements. From needing a sling hoist to get out of bed they gradually built Anton up to managing with a standing hoist, then with a frame. They increased his tolerance for standing, then gradually got him taking steps – initially using a Zimmer frame for support and then progressing to crutches.

Anton's improved mobility meant that he could begin to work on more complex tasks and, for him, cooking was a priority. Once he felt ready he joined the breakfast group, making a full English alongside two other patients. They were joined in our therapy kitchen by occupational therapist Eva and neuropsychologist Monica. The adjustable worktops were lowered to a height that suited wheelchair users and perching stools, and in the bright morning light the group assembled their ingredients.

Cooking is a whole level of complexity up from brushing your teeth. It needs planning, sequencing things in the right order, monitoring your environment and safety awareness – all very much frontal lobe functions. These were tricky for Anton, who would also have to maintain an upright position on his stool while holding a knife or wooden spoon with arms that tended to jerk about. The visual hallucinations had largely settled by now – he joked that the mannequins had taken themselves back to Selfridges – but he still had to concentrate to make sense of what was in front of him.

The previous day Eva had sat down with Anton and made a picture list of the steps he would need to take in order to make scrambled eggs, and he referred to this now. Take the egg from the box, crack it on the edge of the glass bowl (both hands needed for this part), put the shell into the bin, pick up the weighted fork, hold the bowl with his left hand and then beat the eggs. Eva had colour coded the ingredients, taking advantage of Anton's ability to differentiate colours, and he spoke the steps to himself as he went. Next to him, attending to the bacon, was Marge, a chatty older lady with bouffant hair, who gave a running commentary from her wheelchair as if she were watching the 3.10 steeplechase at Aintree. Further along the worktop, Jeff was on toast, a tall and lugubrious man with tufts of grey hair who moved solemnly about the kitchen in complete silence. It was sweaty work, and Anton needed a great deal of 'scaffolding' from the therapists. Before long, though, the smell of cooking bacon began to wind its way down the corridor.

This kind of group work is an essential part of neurorehabilitation. Patients rubbing along together in a joint endeavour has enormous fringe benefits and can cause unexpected shifts in their conditions. The people involved may have a wide range of different impairments, diagnoses, personalities and social backgrounds. But the sense of being in the same boat, albeit more of a leaky rowing boat than a luxury yacht, provides a kind of medical

Dunkirk spirit and much needed emotional support. It allows a retuning of rusty social and communication skills, and observing others with neurological impairments can also help patients to build an understanding of their own.

Anton also attended our Brain Injury Group, four or five patients sitting around a table discussing how the brain works and what can go wrong. He was initially not keen to take part but was gently cajoled by Dennis and soon found himself sitting with the others, chewing the fat. I led a session using a plastic model of the brain to explain to the group which parts do what, and what happens in different kinds of brain injury. More than once during my sessions the pin would come out of the model and the plastic brain would fall to pieces. When I was then unable to reassemble it correctly (it is trickier that you would think) at least one patient would usually tell me it was lucky I am not a brain surgeon. One of my greatest pleasures in this work is to observe the unexpected friendships which often form – the ex-con Essex hard man with the shy Sikh electrician, or the genteel blue-rinse lady with the phone-bound British-Somali teenage girl. These bonds may be strong, and frequently outlive the hospital admission.

Anton worked hard to overcome and adjust to his mixture of cognitive, visual and physical symptoms. Eva began to take him outside and he was able to make his way slowly along the pavement. He rejected the four-wheeled walker in favour of crutches (wobblier but a more acceptable appearance for him) and with a lot of support was able to draw money out of a cash machine. His family began to take him to a local cafe at weekends. Thoughts began to turn to home, and to what sort of life Anton would live once he left us. As well as he was doing, this young inhabitant of the London club scene was still needing some help to go to the loo and get dressed.

*

The question of how (or even why) somebody recovers after an injury to their brain had been bugging me since as a junior doctor I had watched my neurosurgery patient Paul fester in his side-room. I kept thinking of him living out his days in a nursing home (minus his postcard) and it got me wondering how he and others like him ever got better.

When that career detour came to an end I had stumbled blinking out of the fog of sleep deprivation and back into the real world, and I found to my astonishment that I still had friends, family and even (by the skin of my teeth) a girlfriend. Drawn unconsciously to the neurology and stroke wards, I began once again to see patients with brain injuries of one kind or another. Some had impairments as severe as those I had seen in neurosurgery, but here they were receiving regular treatment from therapists. They were being got out of bed, challenged and encouraged to try things out. And, sure enough, some were clearly improving, beginning to use their weak arm or taking tentative steps with support. The contrast with Paul's experience further convinced me that stimulation, practice and exploration are important in recovery. But how did this work? What was going on in these patients' brains that allowed them to regain lost functions?

I came across an intriguing PhD programme: using magnetic brain stimulation to study the return of hand movement after stroke. This seemed to get to the core of the question I was interested in, so I applied. More importantly, the idea of playing with magnets to probe the brain's circuits just sounded plain fun. Before studying patients, though, I would first need to learn a bit about how the healthy brain controls movement. But that should be pretty straightforward – moving your hand is simple. Right?

CHAPTER FOUR

THE BEAUTY OF MOVEMENT

Thomas pulled up in the church car park, switched off the engine and sat to collect his thoughts. He took his typed sermon from his jacket pocket and glanced over it. All Saints' Day was approaching and he wanted to feature St Elizabeth of Hungary. His plan was to draw a contrast between her ministrations to the poor and the UK government's cuts to welfare and support for the vulnerable, quaintly known as austerity. Essentially a moral sermon, he felt, but it mustn't sound too political or preachy. He checked it over once again and was satisfied. He gathered himself up, climbed out and headed up the path through the gusty morning to the entrance. A heavy wind the previous night had brought down the last of the chestnut tree's leaves, and he skidded slightly.

The weak October sun had as yet done nothing for the inside of the church, and although he could not quite see his own breath the pews were pretty icy, so as Thomas turned on the lights he flicked the heaters on too. Having cassocked up in the vestry he rubbed his hands for warmth as the familiar crowd gradually appeared, scattered around the pews. The hubbub slowly built as the chatting got underway, and Thomas got into quite an involved discussion about the previous day's football before remembering that he was supposed to be starting the service. He stepped up to the pulpit, lined up his order of service and Book of Common Prayer and pulled on his reading glasses. Silence descended.

'Grace and peace to you from God our Father and from the Lord Jesus Christ. Amen. Welcome, all, on this gusty morning, and as God brings us autumnal winds from the east let us find warmth in our common worship!'

Thomas let his greeting settle over the pews and as he opened his mouth to continue he became aware of an odd sensation. The whole church seemed to be spinning around him, or, if not, then maybe he had just stepped onto a roundabout. He held onto the pulpit's edge to steady himself and as he did so a cold sweat broke across his brow. He tried to pick up where he had left off but his tongue froze and no words came out. He felt the grip in his hands weakening, and despite his best efforts to cling on he slid to the floor, landing gently on his right side. His feet were stuck in the pulpit and as he looked up at the congregants who were now gathering over him he found that they too seemed to be spinning about. A profound nausea was rising in his head like a terrible wave, and as he looked up again, his friend Andrew's head seemed to be bobbing from side to side. Thomas tried to right himself but now realised that he could not move his arms or legs, which were frozen like blocks of wood on either side of his body. His right arm was possessed of an odd sensation as if it was not really there, and as he lay on the church floor a numb feeling was also creeping down his right leg.

The congregants straightened Thomas up, laid him on one side, in the recovery position, and put a coat under his head. A first-aider was checking his pulse, which seemed to be racing, and he could hear murmurings about calling an ambulance. As the spinning feeling gathered momentum he closed his eyes. He felt as if he were lying on his back just beneath the surface of a pond. As he sank slowly downwards the water's surface and all sound seemed to recede above him. Soon there was only darkness.

*

A man – let's call him Alexander – sits at his breakfast table and contemplates his plate, on which a juicy sausage awaits. He catches a waft of its fried breakfast smell, notices a smear of egg yolk along its side and decides that immediate action is needed. He already has the sausage pinned down with the fork in his left hand and a knife is held in his right: all that remains is to reach out, make a cutting movement and a chunk will be his.

Having decided to take the plunge, Alexander's brain gives the command to reach out and his right arm obeys. The factors that culminate in a decision to move may be several – the smell, a gnawing hunger from his stomach, the visual cue of the sausage in front of him, perhaps the prospect of lunch later that day with a vegetarian aunt. But once the tipping point is reached and the decision made, a complex and well-rehearsed sequence is triggered in order to execute it. Like the US President calling in an air strike by a phone call to the Joint Chiefs, the order is passed on to a large organisation that is primed to do his bidding, freeing up the decision maker to attend to other pressing issues. In Alexander's case that may be the location of the marmalade.

While the process of making the decision is likely to involve several brain regions, the final command to move the arm must leave the brain via a specific area at the top called the primary motor cortex. This is the main exit point for motor commands – motor in the sense of relating to movement – and ultimately controls the arm. To appreciate why a patient with stroke or other brain injury may have difficulty making this movement it is important to understand why most of us can. Lifting the lid on the machinery of movement allows us to approach the problem of what to do when it goes wrong. It also reveals something about why humankind is such a devastatingly successful species.

The human brain is a largely solid lump of cells weighing about three pounds. It consists mainly of neurons – the nerve cells, which do the computing – and glial cells, which provide a supportive scaffolding to maintain them. The neuron is the brain's computational building block. Each one functions as a tiny decision maker in its own right, a logical unit which takes in a large number of inputs and produces just one all-or-nothing output. Either it fires or it does not. Within that modest lump of tissue there are around 100 billion neurons, which are in constant communication with each other via 100 trillion connections, or synapses. Put a vast number of decision-making units in intimate contact with each other, put the whole assembly in control of a living body, and the result is behaviour.

Neurons themselves are highly conserved across species, meaning that from a squid to a rocket scientist evolution has not needed to do much to develop this fundamental building block. They are very specialised to their function, which is to take inputs from several other neighbouring neurons and integrate them into a single output. As a result they are rather different in shape to most cell types found in the body. At the neuron's centre is the cell body. This is chunky and roughly spherical, housing most of the housekeeping machinery – energy supply, waste disposal, etc. From the cell body arise a handful of wispy filament-like projections known as dendrites that are intertwined over a short distance among the neighbouring neurons. These are branched and covered in knobbly spines, so although they are quite short they have a large surface area. The dendrites are the input area and they receive tens of thousands of synapses from other neurons both near and distant. These many inputs are integrated in or near the cell body, and from this projects the long cable-like axon which carries the output.

Depending on the type of neuron the axon may be relatively short or very long indeed. While the cell body is less than a tenth of a millimetre across (and some may be less than a hundredth) the axon may be up to a metre long, making neurons oddly lop-sided cells. At its far end the axon branches into small filaments that pass its output on to many other neurons via their dendrites. In this way the neuron's output is passed along as an electrical message to the next one along the pathway.

Each neuron's many inputs are integrated by electrochemical wizardry into a binary decision: to fire or not to fire. In essence, the neuron's cellular machinery maintains a constant imbalance in the concentration of electrically charged salt molecules – ions of sodium, potassium, chloride and calcium – between the cell's inside and its outside. This means that for each resting neuron there is a small voltage difference across the cell's membrane, negative on the outside and positive on the inside (the membrane is the thin barrier that separates the inside of the cell from the outside world, like the skin of Alexander's sausage). This gradient is actively maintained by millions of tiny channels and pumps studded into the neuron's membrane, working away tirelessly like electrical air-conditioning.

When an inputting neuron fires its synapse onto the receiving neuron's dendrites this has the effect of slightly reversing the voltage gradient. If enough inputting neurons do this at the same time then the overall voltage around the cell body will rise above a certain threshold: this triggers special voltage-sensitive channels to open, causing a flood of current and a transient complete voltage reversal which ripples rapidly down the neuron's axon – an electrical shock wave called an action potential. How this works was figured out by three Cambridge physiologists – Hodgkin, Huxley and Katz – just after the Second World War using giant squid axons, and earned them Nobel prizes. When this neuron 'decided' to fire, all of the many inputting synapses that it receives – some promoting firing, some inhibiting it – were integrated into one output. In this clever way a digital all-or-nothing output was distilled from many inputs.

The action potential will whizz down the nerve's axon all the way to its synapses with the next neurons in the pathway. The axon carrying the output is wrapped along its entire length by a sheath of a substance called myelin, which effectively insulates it from other neurons and allows the action potential to travel fast.

The cerebral cortex is the outer layer of the brain which covers the entire surface of both hemispheres and is made up of the undulating folds that give it its walnut-like appearance. This is the first part that a neurosurgeon sees when they make a hole in the top of the skull and open up the brain's lining, as we had done for Paul. The cortex is made up mainly of grey matter, grey in colour because it contains the neurons' bulky cell bodies. If the neurosurgeon poked their way deeper beneath the surface then the tissue would appear paler: this is the white matter, and contains mainly the axons with their pale myelin sheaths. To use a computing network analogy, the grey matter in the cortex would be the many servers, while the white matter tracts that link them would be the cables. The cortex is where the majority of synapses between neurons occur, and this is where most of the brain's heavy-duty computing power resides.

The final command to move Alexander's right arm must leave the brain from his left primary motor cortex, a long horizontally orientated strip of brain at the rear end of the frontal lobe (just underneath where Stanley Laurel scratches his head). All motor commands to the arm that leave the brain's cortex must pass through here so, as one might imagine, damage to this region from whatever cause results in a loss of movement. These neurons' long axons reach all the way down to the spinal cord, crossing over from left to right as they pass through the bottom of the brain.

Once the axon reaches the level of the spinal cord that it needs to control (in this case in the neck) it forms a synapse there with the second neuron in the pathway, which in turn sends its axon all the way to the relevant arm muscle. This axon's synapses release their neurotransmitter directly onto the muscle's surface and cause it to contract. So the neural pathway all the way from Alexander's motor cortex to his arm consists of just two cells, known rather unimaginatively as the upper and lower motor neurons. The shoulder muscles spring to life, and Alexander's right arm starts to move towards its target.

*

Thomas felt himself rising slowly towards the surface of the pond. He had no idea where he was, and as he tried to open his eyes he found that they were held shut with sticky tape. He tried again and this time they opened, but there was some sort of ointment in them and all he could make out was the bleary outline of a light on a ceiling. He gradually became aware that there was a nurse standing next to him and he tried to say something but discovered that there was a large tube coming out of his mouth. The nurse saw that he was awake and leant over him.

'Hello, Thomas, my name is Evelyn. You are on the Intensive Care Unit at the moment. There is a tube going down into your lungs to help you breathe. You are completely safe but please try not to pull at the tube.'

Thomas looked up at her. She had two heads, which was a little disconcerting. He found that if he looked towards the middle and not to the side then her heads resolved into one again. Above her the square tiles of the suspended false ceiling formed a dizzying grid which stretched away in all directions. If he focused on one tile and fixed on its fake grain he could see that it quivered slightly against its metal bracket, presumably moved by air currents – or was it just his eyes?

'Can you understand what I am saying, Thomas?'

He looked back at Evelyn and nodded, but this head movement brought on the spinning feeling again and with it a wave of nausea.

'That's great! Please do try not to pull at the tubes though.'

He had not been aware of it but his left arm had found its way up to his nose, from which a piece of rubber tubing seemed to be protruding.

Thomas took stock. His right arm and leg did not seem to want to move at all, or only very slightly. He could bend his left knee and even lift that whole leg off the bed. He could lift his left arm up but when he tried to hold it in one place it bobbed and jerked about like a branch in a storm. He tried to screw his eyes shut but could only manage to get them half closed. He could not speak because of the tube in his throat, so he had to wave his left arm about to attract Evelyn's attention. As he did so his arm caught itself in the rails that were keeping Thomas in bed like the sides of a cot. He tried to reposition himself but found that his limbs sank hopelessly into the inflatable mattress, as if he were trying to sit up on a lilo. A plastic pipe by his feet was keeping the mattress topped up with air and would periodically ping. Bleeping in general seemed to be a theme on the ICU, distinctive tones or short phrases set off every time a line was blocked or an infusion finished. As a result, when Thomas closed his eyes and tried to sleep, he found himself floating away on a soundtrack of experimental electronica.

*

The fine control of hand and arm movements is of particular importance to us humans, Alexander included, as it allows us to manipulate our environment. Compared with most animals we have a particularly direct connection between our frontal lobes and our hand muscles, with just two neurons firing in sequence. It is also relatively speedy when compared to other pathways, with large fast-conducting axons. This is by no means the only connection from the brain to the muscles: there are other less direct pathways, for example via the brainstem or via intermediary neurons in the spinal cord. In fact the existence of a direct and fast output from the motor cortex to the spinal motor neurons is unique to dexterous primates, and presumably reflects the importance that evolution has given to precise control by the brain of the hand.

A similarly direct connection is seen also to the muscles of the face and mouth but not to those of the trunk and legs. As the emergence of complex language and speech is arguably our biggest evolutionary advantage over other species it is perhaps not surprising that the muscles responsible should also be favoured in this way. In macaques it is possible to separate out the 'old' (in an evolutionary sense) regions of the primary motor cortex, whose projections reach the spinal cord indirectly, from the 'newer' direct connection. In developing dexterous hand control and speech, evolution has seemingly grafted a new and more advanced system on top of the old one.

As Alexander reaches out with his knife several other muscles must kick in. If we tried to reach our arm out without any adjustments then we would topple forward. This does not happen because our trunk and back muscles automatically contract to stabilise our core and offset the shift in our gravitational centre. The motor cortex does not have to worry about this, however, and in fact is not necessary at all for these stabilising movements to take place: they are largely taken care of lower down, in the circuits of the lower brainstem and spinal cord. Odd as it may seem, many quite complex movements can be made without the brain being involved at all. The most dramatic example is perhaps the headless chicken who continues to run around the farmyard. A 'decerebrate cat', who has had a cut made that effectively separates the bottom of the brainstem from the spinal cord, can make fully formed stepping movements with its legs, and the same is true of a 'spinal cat' in which the spinal cord has been cut lower down (these experiments were done in the 1920s so please don't firebomb my house).

We all know, if we think about it, that limb movements can be generated without conscious thought. The automatic pulling away of an arm from a hot stove, for example, or a knee jerk elicited by an enthusiastic doctor with a reflex hammer. In both cases the sensory input from a limb causes a muscle contraction via a single synapse in the spinal cord, entirely independently of the brain. Current thinking suggests that the spinal cord contains circuits that act as pattern generators, and that these can make fairly complicated rhythmic movements, such as walking, with little or no input from the brain. It is harder to prove that such spinal pattern generators exist in humans, and in people with spinal cord injuries we do not see automatic walking movements. But this illustrates the generally accepted idea that there is a hierarchy of motor control from fully automatic to conscious and deliberate: the humble knee jerk at one end, and 'I Have a Dream' at the other, with Alexander's breakfast presumably somewhere in the middle.

So the evolution of complex movement in humans is a story of the gradual domination of older motor circuits in the lower brain and spinal cord by an increasingly sophisticated and bossy cerebral cortex sitting on top. You can even witness this process in action as children grow. When a paediatrician assesses a newly born baby (or if they are stuck for a party trick) they will sometimes dangle them upright with a foot touching the bed, which triggers a rhythmic stepping movement resembling walking. If they are really going to town (and the parent is not watching) they may sit the baby up and then suddenly drop it backwards. This causes the baby to spread its arms quickly outwards and then back in again: the Moro reflex. Both of these movements are 'primitive' reflexes and they reflect how extraordinarily unfinished we humans are when we pop out of the womb. Compare us to newborn cattle, who just stand up and get on with it. We have to come out at least three months early – sent before our time into this breathing world scarce half made up – because any longer in the womb and our outsized heads would get stuck. From an evolutionary perspective our transient helplessness as newborns is presumably offset by the advanced trickery that our burgeoning bonces concoct later on.

As a baby grows, its developing cerebral cortex begins to kick in and gradually asserts its authority over the spinal cord and lower brain. As a result both of these reflexes usually disappear by the time the child is three to six months old: evolution in real time. These primitive reflexes can reappear later. The circuits which mediate them are still there, and as the cortex's influence wanes they may be released from their top-down suppression. If you examine a patient in whom the cerebral hemispheres have largely ceased to function, for example with Creutzfeldt-Jacob disease or very advanced Alzheimer's disease, then you can demonstrate a grasp reflex (automatically grabbing onto a finger placed in the palm) or a rooting response (turning the mouth toward a touch on the cheek to seek the breast).

As Alexander reaches out with his knife his primary motor cortex is calling the shots. An illustration in humans of the map showing how parts of this strip of cortex correspond to the body parts they control produces the 'homunculus', or little man. This figure has enormous lips and cheeks, a tiny neck, huge hands and little legs, a grotesque distortion reflecting the relative importance of these body parts. This motor map can be examined in detail by stimulating the motor cortex and seeing what happens, either directly in animals or indirectly in humans using a focused pulse from a magnetic coil held over the scalp. This can also be demonstrated directly in humans during awake craniotomies, an operation to remove a tumour sitting close to an important area of cortex. The patient lies on the operating table with their cerebral cortex exposed and is asked to do something while the operation progresses – to speak, for example, or in a recent London case to play a violin. The surgeon meanwhile stimulates the cortical area in question in order to check what function would be lost if that region were excised.

But how does the cortex 'know' which muscles to activate for a given movement? There are more than thirty-five muscles in the arm and hand, each with its own nerve supply. To straighten the arm, for example, Alexander will need to use the triceps muscle. He also needs some of the shoulder's rotator cuff muscles to bring the arm forward, the finger flexors to grip the knife, the wrist flexors and extensors to stabilise the wrist, and another muscle to keep his index finger out. As the reaching movement progresses the pattern and roles of these muscles will also change.

If each output neuron in the primary motor cortex were linked simply to an individual muscle then a reach-and-grasp movement would present a hideously complex engineering challenge, but the system is cleverer than that. Individual output neurons (known as 'pyramidal cells' on account of their shape) encode *movements*, or aspects of movements, rather than the muscles themselves. In monkeys, for example, around half of the pyramidal cells encode the direction of movement of a body part in space. This directional characteristic holds regardless of the actual muscles needed to make the movement in the monkey's current position, adjusting for example if the monkey were facing in another direction.

Other pyramidal neurons encode different aspects of the movement, such as force or speed. So although the primary motor cortex as the common exit point is hierarchically the 'lowest' of the brain regions concerning movement, there seems already to be a degree of abstraction at that level: the properties of the desired movement, rather than the individual muscles needed to make it, are represented here. The process of taking the desired direction of movement and translating that into an actual pattern of muscles seems to take place lower down, probably in the spinal cord.

So if the primary motor cortex is the final exit point for a motor command to leave the brain, where does the command actually originate? There are several 'higher' motor regions in the brain, mostly in the frontal lobes sitting forward of the primary motor cortex: together these make up the cortical motor network. Making a movement typically involves activity in many or most of these higher motor regions, and Alexander's are firing away as he reaches out. It seems that the further 'upstream' of the primary motor cortex you get, the more complex and abstract is the movement which is represented.

Some of what we know about these regions comes from patients with epileptic seizures. These occur when the electrical activity in part of the brain gets out of control, and neurons which usually fire individually start to discharge rhythmically and in synchrony. Often the seizure spreads quickly to encompass much or all of the brain's cortex, leading to unconsciousness and violent convulsions. If, however, the seizure remains confined to one part of the brain – a focal seizure – then a specific symptom will arise that relates to that region's function, as it fires repeatedly.

A seizure in the primary motor cortex causes rhythmic jerking of the relevant body part. As the runaway electrical activity works its way sideways along the motor strip the jerking migrates relentlessly down from the face to the arm and then the leg – this is named the Jacksonian march (for the Victorian neurologist Hughlings Jackson). A seizure confined to the supplementary motor area causes a fixed rigid posturing of the limbs in a fencing position, with one arm held flexed and the other outstretched. Further forward in the frontal lobes a seizure may cause quite complex movements, such as cycling motions with the legs or even getting up and rushing about the room.

These seizure patterns support the idea that the further forward in the frontal lobes you get, the more complex and abstracted the movement representation seems to be. The idea then is that a motor command starts somewhere near the front as an abstract idea and works its way backwards to the primary motor cortex, becoming progressively encoded as specifics of the planned movement as it goes.

You could argue that asking where in the brain a command to make a movement originates is somewhat meaningless: depending on how far up the chain of command you want to look, you would find its origin diffusely in all of the external cues, internal thoughts and even emotional factors that gave rise to the desire to make the action in the first place. I mentioned at the start of this chapter the motivators for Alexander's reaching movement: the smell of breakfast, the sight of egg yolk and the dreadful prospect of nut roast for lunch. Add to that perhaps the sound of sizzling bacon (temporal lobe) provoking anticipation of the taste (insular cortex), and even an emotional response to those cues (limbic system). One might suggest that the reaching movement originated in any or all of the relevant brain regions.

*

Soon after Thomas woke up on the ICU his wife Gail appeared at his side. She kissed his forehead and clutched his stronger left hand, tears of relief in her eyes. She told him what had happened, supported by one of the doctors. Thomas had slipped into a coma on the way to the hospital so when he arrived the doctors had inserted a tube into his trachea and put him on a breathing machine. Once Thomas was stabilised the doctors had done a CT brain scan. This showed blood at the bottom of the brain, in the part of the brainstem known as the pons. It was not yet clear why he had bled, but initial scans of the arteries had not shown anything unusual and it may just have been due to high blood pressure. The bleed was on the left side so this meant that his right arm and leg were weak, though his left side was not moving normally either. Unfortunately it had also interfered with several other important structures. His eye movements were not aligned, hence the double-headed nurse. His face was weak on both sides, which was why he could not fully close his eyes. The connections to his cerebellum were damaged, so the movement on his stronger left side was poorly coordinated. It was too early to know for sure, but the part of the brainstem that controls the tongue, larynx and pharynx was probably also affected. This meant that speaking would likely be difficult and he might not be able to swallow normally.

As Thomas listened to this grim analysis Gail held a laminated chart in front of him so that he could interject or ask questions. This included 'Yes', 'No' and the letters of the alphabet. Thomas raised his wobbly left arm and started jabbing away at it.

'S–O– [space] W–H–A–T– [space] I–S– [space] T–H–E– [space] B–A–D– [space] N–E–W–S– ?'

Gail laughed through tears of relief at this joke and at the line of communication which had now been opened. On the plus side, all of the higher brain areas appeared intact so Thomas's thinking skills were likely to be relatively unscathed.

Over the next weeks they changed the tube in his trachea to a tracheostomy – this is a smaller tube that comes out of a hole in your neck rather than your mouth – and changed the feeding tube in his nose for a smaller one that went straight into his stomach. They managed to get him off the breathing machine entirely and onto a normal ward. Gail was by Thomas's side almost constantly, and between her and their teenage girls they did their best to keep his spirits up. But this man with a mission and a calling was entirely beached. For now he was bed-bound with a hole in his neck, one tube in his stomach and another in his willy. He had little control of his bodily functions and needed everything doing for him.

Thomas was an intelligent man and he realised that his life would never again be the same.

*

Alexander must be ravenous by now but salvation is in sight. His knife has finally reached its target and is pressed against the top of the sausage, ready to cut. How does he know how hard to press down and to saw back and forth? He has cut a sausage before, so he knows that it will need more force than cutting through butter but not as much as cutting a raw carrot. The internal model of the world that he has been building up over the years therefore gives him a rough starting point, but it is likely not to be that accurate. What if this sausage is one of those dense venison ones? He doesn't want to clink his knife on the plate by going through too hard but equally he would like his breakfast sometime soon. This is where he will use the feedback he receives from his muscles and joints, and from vision, which will guide him as the cutting progresses.

Running parallel to the primary motor cortex, just behind it in the parietal lobe, is its counterpart for sensation. The primary sensory cortex is the first staging post for sensory information arriving in the cerebral cortex from the outside world: here the flow is inwards not outwards. Just as we have a motor homunculus in front we likewise have a sensory homunculus behind, and the face, mouth and hands are again over-represented. Sensation comes in a number of modalities, with receptors in our body for each – pain, temperature, vibration, muscle stretch, joint position sense – and all can be used to inform our model of the outside world and to guide movements.

The neurons in the sensory cortex send projections mainly backwards into the parietal lobe, for the sensations arriving from below to be processed and analysed. However, they also send copies of some of this information forwards to their equivalent regions in the neighbouring primary motor cortex – sensory thumb to motor thumb, sensory fingertip to motor fingertip. This allows feedback from the arm Alexander is moving to make adjustments to the movement as it takes place, a process called sensorimotor integration.

This is probably not in itself enough to guarantee a clean cut and no plate clink. The problem is the time lag. If having given a command to move we had to wait for the resulting sensory information to come back from the limb before making an adjustment – a round trip of forty or fifty milliseconds – then the movement would not be that smooth and the arm would oscillate to and fro.

How much more efficient it would be if instead we had a system that could predict the likely outcome of a movement *as we make it* – an internal model that calculated the likely sensory feedback that a given movement would generate. We could then compare the predicted feedback to the actual feedback once it arrives, and if there is any difference we could use this to refine our model. What I am describing here is a feed-forward system. We are more familiar with feedback systems: think of old-school central heating with a boiler and a thermostat. You set the temperature you would like, and if the temperature is below this then the boiler comes on. The room temperature gradually climbs, and once the thermostat reaches the target temperature it switches the boiler off again. There is then a slow oscillation around the desired temperature.

If instead your super-intelligent heating system knew the outside weather conditions, whether anyone had left any windows open (my son, for example), how many people were in the rooms at that moment and if the cat flap was working properly, it could make a prediction about how long to switch on for. The model could then 'learn' and improve its accuracy by checking the outcome against its prediction. This would result in better predictions and much less in the way of temperature fluctuations. This is a feed-forward system. In a movement context such a system might estimate the force needed to pick up a suitcase based on an expectation of its likely weight. If the suitcase turns out to be empty – and we bump ourselves on the nose as a result – then the discrepancy from what was expected could allow our prediction model to be adjusted for the next attempt.

It just so happens that we have a highly effective and specialised feed-forward device to smooth out our movements: the cerebellum, which sits neatly at the back of the brain like a performance-enhancing afterthought. It resembles a butterfly-shaped wedge, and if you look closely you can see hundreds of tiny horizontal folds on its surface, with a thin worm-like vertical ridge in the middle. Cut through the middle and you would see a delicate tree-like internal structure, a little like broccoli only much more fine. Look under a microscope and you would see that its entire cortex consists of a repeating arrangement of neurons that is so beautifully regular as to be almost crystalline.

Its small lobes are highly unusual for the brain, not only in their hyper-regular internal structure but also in the circuitry itself. Most neuronal circuits include a mish-mash of reciprocal connections, with feedback loops, multiple inputs and multiple outputs. The cerebellum has relatively few feedback connections and only one effective output pathway. Its output neurons, the Purkinje cells, also have a very odd balance of inputs: each one receives synapses from around 100,000 of one input type (the mossy fibres) but from just one of the other (climbing fibres).

This curious arrangement puzzled neuroscientists for years, until a prodigious young Cambridge physiologist produced an elegant theory as part of his PhD thesis. David Marr saw the cerebellum's unusual structure and connections as being perfect for it to act as a learning machine to improve the smoothness of movement. He suggested that as the motor cortex sends off a motor command to the muscles it sends a copy of the command in parallel to the cerebellum, which generates a prediction as to what sort of sensory feedback that movement should generate. The cerebellum also receives a rich constant flow of live sensory input: any mismatch between the real and predicted inputs generates a strong error signal to the Purkinje cell, adjusting the predictive model. The result of this arrangement is that we have a good idea of the consequences of any planned movement as we make it, and long before we receive the resulting feedback.

As a result, we are able to make corrections more quickly than would otherwise be possible. When picking up a known weight between thumb and index finger, for example, we do not need to wait for sensory feedback from our hands to apply the correct force. Likewise, as we move an object across a trajectory the load force varies, but the adjustments in grip force are made so precisely and quickly that it can only be explained by use of an internal model.

This idea of taking a copy of an action and predicting the likely result is known as 'efferent copy', and it pops up elsewhere in neuroscience. As a general principle we need to be able to screen out the consequences of our own actions if we are to remain sensitive to external stimuli. It is thought that crickets do this when they strigulate (rub their legs together – my father-in-law's favourite word), otherwise the loud noise they make would render them deaf to nearby sounds and therefore vulnerable. A copy of the motor command is used to predict the resulting sound which is then subtracted from what they hear: biological noise-cancelling headphones. We do the same when we talk, sending an efferent copy of the planned speech to our auditory areas, so that we can distinguish our speech from that of somebody else. Efferent copy is probably also the reason that we are unable to tickle ourselves.

Tickling is by its nature unpredictable: if we already have a copy of the sensation that will result then no amount of armpit auto-tickling will make you wriggle.

David Marr's theory of the cerebellum remains as elegant as ever fifty years on. But his idea in 1969 was also important ultimately in giving rise to the whole field of computational neuroscience. The following year, 1970, he published a theory of the neocortex and in 1971 a theory of the hippocampus, before then developing a theory of visual processing that now forms the basis of some forms of artificial intelligence. Not a bad few years' work for one person and compared by some to Einstein's flurry of world-changing papers in 1905. Marr's death from leukaemia at the age of thirty-five robbed neuroscience of one of its greats.

*

It took a long time for Thomas to stabilise. Having made it from ICU to the regular ward he then developed pneumonia and had to return there, as his poorly coordinated swallow would send his own saliva down the wrong way and onto his chest. It was almost Christmas by the time his breathing and swallow were stable enough for his tracheostomy to be removed. As a result he now had a voice again but this only revealed the extent of his speech difficulty. Just as his limbs were poorly coordinated, the same was true of his tongue and speech apparatus, so his words were not only slurred but burst out in an unpredictable torrent.

By the time Thomas arrived on our rehabilitation unit he was more than four months in and his spirits were sagging. There were signs of improvement in some respects but he remained entirely dependent. His right arm and leg were now moving better, but he had little fine motor control and with a poorly functioning cerebellum all his movements were very jerky. The cerebellum can be thought of as the graphics card of movement

– without it the graphics on your PC still work more or less, but they are pretty clunky. He still had the double vision and the facial weakness. He still needed the feeding tube in his stomach for all of his nutrition. He needed a sling hoist to get him out of bed and a special tilting chair to sit out safely.

The physiotherapists spent days and weeks working with Thomas to strengthen his trunk, allowing him gradually to correct his tendency to slump to his right when seated, and eventually we were able to sit him at a table in our day room in a standard chair. The physios began to stand him up, which was exhausting to start with and his movements were too unpredictable for him to take any steps. But even if he was unable to walk he was absolutely determined to be able to stand up at a table.

Thomas spent hours with our speech therapists and they re-trained his swallow, working on improving strength (blowing into a straw against resistance) and drilling the relevant tongue movements. He began to take a little food orally, only purée to start with, but this was gradually built up and after around three months we were able to remove the tube from his stomach. Feeding himself was difficult, as his stronger left arm struggled to hold a fork steady, but after intensive training using weighted cutlery he began to manage.

Thomas slowly regained a degree of control over his speech apparatus – you had to listen carefully but once you got your ear in you could understand most of what he was saying. He had to concentrate intensely on each word and phrase to get it out: the equivalent difference perhaps between walking normally across a room and stumbling across a wobbly rowing boat while carrying a tray of glasses with one hand. As Thomas began to communicate more effectively it became clear why he was so keen to stand up at a table: he was intending to hold services and to preach. This meant standing up at a pulpit. We began increasingly to get a sense not only of his sharp intellect and philosophical bent – he had a doctorate in history – but also of his steely determination. He was not going to let a bit of blood around the brainstem prevent him from fulfilling his calling.

*

Success – the sausage cutting has begun and is going smoothly! While the knife in Alexander's right hand saws away, the fork in his left keeps the sausage pinned down. To keep his breakfast from sliding about he must apply a degree of force through the fork which varies with each change of pressure through the knife. This is a classic bimanual task: the two hands must cooperate for things to go smoothly.

At first glance the brain's two hemispheres look physically separate, with a large chasm running front to back between them. In fact they are joined at the bottom of this fissure by a long flat strip of white matter – the corpus callosum – which is a thick band of projections linking many cortical regions to their equivalents on the other side. This bridge between the brain's two halves would seem to be crucial, but in fact the two hemispheres can function without it remarkably well. Some people are born without a corpus callosum at all and seem to manage fine, though their brains will of course develop differently.

Rarely in the treatment of epilepsy it is necessary to remove the corpus callosum surgically – a callosotomy – to stop seizures spreading from one hemisphere to the other. In such 'split brain' patients there is little noticeable effect of what sounds like a drastic procedure, and old reports of a patient's left hand doing one thing while their right hand wrestles to stop it are probably exaggerated. But for functions which are largely or completely specialised to one side or the other, such as language (left), number calculations (left) or visuospatial processing (right), you can detect a failure of the two halves to communicate. When such a patient is blindfolded then handed an object such as a toothbrush they are reportedly able to name it if it is held in the right hand but not the left hand. This is presumably because the sensory information from the left hand is processed in the right hemisphere and once there cannot access the language regions on the left. Similarly, when a simple mathematical sum is presented to just one side of a patient's visual field they have no difficulty if it is shown to the right (left visual cortex) but perform no better than chance if it is shown to the left.

If callosotomy patients are asked to perform a continuous movement with both hands, such as tracing circles with a pen in each hand, then the synchronisation breaks down and their hands get out of synch. Conversely, they perform better than control subjects in tasks where conflicting spatial representations on each side of the brain would normally interfere with each other: they have no difficulty rubbing their tummy while patting their head, for example. But as Alexander cuts his sausage the two halves of his brain are certainly talking to each other, integrating all sorts of sensory information from one arm into the forces generated by the other.

Alexander's battle with his breakfast has got us into a whole lot of motor neuroscience and he has still not eaten. If this were a restaurant he might by now be trying to catch the waiter's eye or considering making a run for it. In fact we have barely scratched the surface, but some of what is going on under the bonnet should now be apparent. But why the major focus on movement? What has this got to do with recovery from brain injury?

Movement is our only way of interacting with the world. This may be by typing, by spearing a fish to avoid starvation, by holding the hand of someone you love, or by raising a quizzical eyebrow in the manner of Roger Moore. Even complex language requires advanced motor control to express it.

To understand how we move is to understand much about the brain in general. The cerebellum models our movements, but in fact the brain is constantly modelling all aspects of the world around us, using a combination of previous experience and current sensory information to make predictions about what will happen next. This real-time modelling of the world is so fundamental to our conscious experience that at times the model itself becomes our perceived reality: we are effectively living in the world as we expect to find it. In the context of brain injury and recovery this can give rise to some odd paradoxes, and nowhere more so perhaps than in the visual system.

Mostly, though, the disruption of movement after stroke or other brain injury is particularly disabling. If you ask a patient who has recently had a stroke what it is that they would most like to change the answer almost always relates to movement: standing, walking, using my hand. But it is not all doom and gloom. At the risk of sounding like a Bible salesman I would like to give you some good news: the brain has a truly extraordinary capacity for reorganisation and recovery in the face of damage. The extent of this capacity has only been appreciated and understood over recent years and it raises questions about how we should treat patients after an event like a stroke.

Over the months he spent with us Thomas fought his way back to many of the functions he had lost, though by no means all. When I think of all the neural processes that have to go smoothly in Alexander's intact brain for him to cut that sausage I conversely wonder how he would manage to do anything at all if the systems involved were damaged. Armed with this knowledge I marvel at Thomas regaining the ability to sit up at a table and feed himself. Not only this but, before long, and through sheer force of character, he had us all sitting downstairs in the hospital chapel fully in thrall to his intensity of purpose.

When the time came for him to leave hospital Thomas returned to the house he shared with Gail, a small vicarage which fortunately was wheelchair accessible and could take some adaptations.

This in itself was a fairly miraculous outcome – many had expected him to be discharged to a nursing home. But Thomas was already making plans for a future return to his previous duties, his impressive recovery resulting in large part from his determination to get his life back. But it would not be possible without a combination of the brain's innate recovery mechanisms and a prolonged period of work by a team of highly skilled professionals.

So how does this work? What is happening in the brain to make it possible? I am next going to consider what we have learned recently about neuroplasticity. And I promise, no more sausages.

CHAPTER FIVE

THE PLASTIC BRAIN

Claire had not spoken for over a year. She was in her late thirties, a mother of three young children and by all accounts a live wire. Her quick wit was a byword among her family and friends, and before her illness she would always be the one to make a party go with a bang. Her partner brought in a short video she had made the month before her collapse. She had been training as a counsellor and in it she was practising a presentation on the importance of communication skills, something which clearly came naturally to her. She spoke directly to camera and bobbed about, a little ball of animation whose hands gesticulated and whose wavy brown hair flicked from side to side as she talked. Something in her small features subverted the serious points she was making as she intermixed jokes with her talk and shot conspiratorial glances at the viewer. It was sincere and captivating.

Her love of a good time had probably been a factor in Claire's illness. On an evening out with friends a few drinks had led to a few more, and then to some cocaine to keep the night going. An aneurysm just beneath her brain ruptured, a blister-like weakness in one of the large arteries spilling blood into and around her frontal lobes. She collapsed immediately, and the swelling of the affected brain was such that when the neuro-surgeons operated to put a metal clip on the leaking aneurysm they also had to remove a section of her skull on both sides. This left Claire with a plate-sized gap in the bone, so that the scalp sagged disconcertingly inward above her eyes and behind her hairline.

By the time Claire joined our ward her skull had been repaired with a metal plate, but this did not of course fix the injury to the brain itself. On her scans I could see scarring and extensive damage to the frontal lobes on both sides, particularly the folds that sit just above the eyes. There was also patchy involvement of her motor areas, particularly on the right. She had spent many months on intensive care at her local hospital and when we accepted her for rehabilitation the reports suggested that although she had regained consciousness she remained very impaired.

Claire arrived from the referring hospital on a stretcher and once she had been hoisted onto one of our beds we could see that she was partially curled up in a ball, her legs bent up at the hips and knees. Her hair was gathered up into a bun and her usually bright eyes were flat and expressionless. When Dennis and I introduced ourselves she made eye contact but showed no other response. I asked her to close her eyes, to see whether she could understand a simple instruction, and she was able to. As I moved on to the rest of the examination she kept on closing her eyes, as if she were stuck on my first instruction. She was able to move her right arm and could use it to some extent but her left arm and both legs were entirely immobile. I could stretch her legs out from their flexed position but as I relaxed my grip they were pulled straight back in again by strong involuntary muscle activity. It was like trying to string a longbow in reverse.

Claire held a pencil tightly in her right hand and we knew

that she could write a few words. I told her my name and that I was one of the doctors. She looked down at her piece of paper and wrote 'doctors doctors doctors'. She could write 'yes' and 'no' in response to simple questions, so we were able to establish that she knew she was in hospital but not which one. She was unclear on the month but knew she had had a bleed on the brain. When I asked if she had any questions she wrote 'questions questions questions' and then her writing tailed slowly off into a wiggly line. In this pathological repeating of words and actions Claire was showing evidence of perseveration, a feature typical of this pattern of damage, which is a failure of the frontal lobes' function in keeping our actions moving along a sequence. Affected people will often get stuck on one step. Despite my best efforts I was unable to coax Claire into any speech at all, and although her limited writing provided her with a basic means to answer questions, she could not initiate any communication.

Claire showed an assortment of severe and interacting neurological impairments rendering her entirely helpless and dependent on nursing care. The referring hospital had not so far been able to offer her much in the way of therapy input and, from the descriptions given in the notes, her condition had been largely static for some months now. The question for us was whether an intensive therapy programme at this relatively late stage would change anything.

*

Neuroplasticity is the brain's capacity to remould its connections and behaviour in response to prior experience. Our brains' many networks are composed of distinct regions joined by neural pathways. In each pathway information passes along a sequence of neurons, one connected to the next by an electrochemical synapse. With tens of billions of neurons sitting in a dense mesh one might imagine such a pathway as a track winding through a thick and impenetrable forest, hard to perceive at first but easier to find when well trodden.

The earliest and perhaps most obvious form of plasticity is seen as we grow and develop. We recognise instinctively that a child's early experiences play a role in determining how they turn out, that while genetic factors are important our exposure to life also leaves an imprint which affects how we function in adulthood. What is less obvious is the extent to which such factors affect the physical development of the brain. This was first apparent from a set of classic experiments in the 1960s looking at how the cat's visual system develops.

As it does for us, the processing of visual information for the cat takes place right at the back of the brain, just above the nape of the neck in the cortex of the occipital lobes. Information from the retinas enters the brain through the optic nerve and crosses to the opposite side to synapse in a relay station near the centre. From there projections reach up and back to the primary visual cortex – this is where visual processing begins.

If you record electrical activity from individual neurons in an adult cat's visual cortex many cells will have a strong preference for left or right, responding primarily to a flash of light given into that eye. The sides to which the neurons respond are not randomly intermixed but are arranged in neat stripes – ocular dominance columns. But far from being predetermined it turns out that this tidy arrangement depends on the conditions in which the cat has been reared. If it has had no visual input at all – if the poor cat has been kept in the dark from birth – then these columns do not form. If instead the normal pattern is allowed to develop but then one eye is covered up within a few months of birth something quite odd happens. Neurons which were previously dominant for the now-covered eye start to respond instead to the uncovered eye. Not only that, but those neurons quickly lose the ability to respond to the covered eye at all – within a week or so there is even a physical peeling-back of the neurons reaching up to the cortex from the lower regions on the deprived side but not from the other. This effect is only seen if the eye is covered within the first few months of life – during which it can be reversed if the eye is re-exposed – but not later.

This re-wiring in response to covering one eye is called ocular dominance plasticity, and the fact that it is only seen within the first months of development suggests there is a 'critical period' for this form of plasticity. During this window there seems to be a process of active competition between the two eyes for the prime real estate of visual cortex. Each side's pathway depends on continuing external stimulation to maintain its territory and the neurons will shrink back if it loses it – the input received from the outside world is physically moulding the brain's projections.

The importance of receiving a correct visual input is not confined to cats. In fact anybody who has one lazy eye from a missed childhood squint has undergone a similar process – if one eye is not correctly aligned during the critical period then visual function from the affected eye never fully develops. Tantalisingly, this form of early plasticity can be reactivated much later: applying a disinhibiting drug to the brain's surface in adult rats seems to reawaken the potential for ocular dominance plasticity, suggesting that inhibitory circuits within the cortex itself are actively suppressing it.

We also see a critical period for plasticity in the effects of damage to the developing brain in children. Rasmussen's encephalitis is a truly horrid but fortunately very rare condition in children, usually under the age of ten, in which one of their brain's two hemispheres gradually stops working and shrinks. Over a few months they not only lose all of the functions on that side of the brain but also develop constant and intractable epileptic seizures arising from the affected regions. Why this should happen is still not clear, but the relentless atrophy proves largely resistant to all medication and forms of treatment. The epilepsy is so severe that in some cases the only way to stop it is almost unthinkable – to surgically remove that entire hemisphere.

This is clearly a horrific consideration and done only as a last resort in an already terrible situation. Performed in an adult a hemispherectomy would lead to severe and permanent disability. You can in fact preview what this would be like by temporarily 'freezing' half of the brain, and my colleagues used to do this when I was a junior doctor. This sounds like a twisted neurological party trick but was actually part of the battery of tests for adults who were being considered for epilepsy surgery. Targeted surgery is in fact extremely effective in stopping seizures in some patients but you must be entirely sure you will not render somebody unable to speak as a result. Almost all right-handed people (and even most left-handed people) do the bulk of their language processing in the left hemisphere, but with epilepsy surgery there is no room for doubt. These days we use functional MRI scans to locate the language centres, but before this was available the procedure was rather more drastic and involved injecting an anaesthetic called sodium amobarbital directly into the internal carotid artery on one side of the neck. The patient would be asked to keep both arms up in the air and to count backwards from thirty: as the drug kicked in one arm would slump to their side and half of their face would droop. If that side was dominant for language then the counting and all speech would stop and you would have your answer. This is effectively a temporary stroke and for a few minutes the patient would be entirely incapacitated. The effects would gradually wear off and then half an hour later you would do the other side. This is definitely not for the faint-hearted, but then nor is undergoing brain surgery.

In children with Rasmussen's, whose median age at onset is six, a left hemispherectomy abolishes the seizures in the majority but there is also an immediate and complete loss of speech. Within a few weeks, however, they begin to be able to distinguish some words again. By one year post-surgery most children can repeat words and even engage in simple conversation at a level that is better than before the operation. Their language processing must therefore have been taken on to some extent by the right hemisphere. This is not to say that cortical regions previously specialised for other functions have now been repurposed for language – we know that the language network spans both hemispheres, especially in children – but, rather, the use of an existing wider network has shifted in response to the change. We do not see such a dramatic extent of spontaneous reorganisation in adults and this is presumably because the child's brain is still developing at the time of the surgery.

As a trainee I remember being amazed to meet an eighteen-year-old girl in the neurology clinic who had effectively lost most of her left hemisphere in a stroke at the age of eleven. She had been lying with her neck bent over the back of the sofa, in a prolonged state of holiday boredom as children often are (or were before phones), but in doing so she had twisted a carotid artery and blocked off her left anterior circulation. She became mute, lost all power on her right side and was in hospital for months. Seven years later and the scan still looked horrific – essentially the front two thirds of her left hemisphere was shrunken scar tissue. And yet there she was chatting away to me. She had a degree of learning difficulty but was essentially able to function. Her right arm was still fairly weak but she was entirely independent getting about. Clearly her developing brain had now established some of what had been mainly left hemisphere functions, including language, on the right side.

As we have developed more sophisticated techniques to study how the brain's functions are laid out we can now appreciate more subtle effects of development in healthy humans. The regions of the motor cortex given over to controlling individual digits of either hand – their cortical representations – can be mapped out using magnetic stimulation. Studying blind adults who are highly proficient in Braille you find that the index finger of their reading hand has a much larger representation than that of the non-reading hand – larger also than the equivalent in blind adults who do not use Braille – at the expense of a smaller area for their little finger. Similarly, the overall size of the non-dominant hand's representation is greater in keyboard players than in non-musicians, while the posterior hippocampus (which stores spatial or navigational memories) is enlarged in London's taxi drivers – famous for having to memorise thousands of streets and shortcuts – as compared either to non-drivers or to bus drivers. So it seems that our brains' structure and layout can be moulded by experience not only during development but also in adulthood.

The examples I have given to this point would perhaps suggest that neuroplasticity is something which takes place gradually over a long period or during development – some call this structural plasticity. In fact neuroscience abounds also with examples of rapid changes in brain organisation, either in response to a change in circumstances or during the process of learning – so-called functional plasticity. Some years ago I visited Gerald Finnerty, a neuroscientist at King's College London who had observed this directly. He worked with rats and was interested particularly in their whiskers, which are crucial in allowing them to feel their way around tight spaces. The input from each whisker is processed in its own region of the rats' sensory cortex – if you vibrate the corresponding whisker then those neurons fire – where their representations are laid out in neat rows, like the paving stones of a particularly tidy patio. This sensory map is often called the barrel cortex, resembling neatly stacked barrels in a distillery.

Finnerty showed that interfering with the rat's whiskers caused rapid shifts in how the barrel cortex was organised. Having made his cortical map he would trim one whisker short, effectively preventing it from functioning, and then release the rat back into its maze. Re-examining the barrel cortex after a few days he would find that the barrel which had been deprived of its input had begun instead to respond to neighbouring intact whiskers. If instead he destroyed one of the barrels in the cortex itself then the disconnected whisker would develop representations in neighbouring regions. He showed that this reorganisation resulted from changes within the synapses of neurons linking the adjacent barrels. So the topographical layouts of the brain's sensory maps, far from being fixed, are fluid and are moulded according to their interactions with the outside world. You can demonstrate a similar effect in humans, recording small electrical fields over the scalp to stake out cortical sensory maps. Numbing the subject's thumb and forefinger with local anaesthetic causes representations of neighbouring digits to appear in that part of the cortex within minutes.

We can also see rapid shifts in how the cortex is organised as a response to learning a new skill. If you were to map out a rat's motor cortex and then train it to reach its forelimb through a hole for a pellet you would find that these motor maps shift in response. The representation of the trained forelimb would grow in size after ten days of training, encroaching on neighbouring representations in the process. Once you stopped the training that limb's representation would shrink back down to baseline within a week. A similar effect is seen in monkeys, and while you cannot of course apply such techniques to humans you can use functional MRI scanning to identify which brain regions are active while we perform a task. Moving a finger involves firing up the hand area of our primary motor cortex and this is visible on the scan. If you train somebody to make a specific sequence of finger movements as quickly as possible then soon their performance of the learned sequence improves. If you scan their brain while they do it, comparing pre- and post-training, you see a large activity increase in the motor cortex during the learned sequence but not during an unlearned sequence. This difference lasts for several months after the end of training and presumably reflects changes in how the brain is executing that movement having learned it.

In all mammals studied with similar experiments we see such shifts in cortical maps in response to changes in the world around us, indicating that the organisation of the brain's cortex is far from fixed and instead reflects a dynamic interpretation of our environment. There is no evidence to suggest that regions of cortex can take on entirely different roles or be repurposed for new functions – the brain's many specialised networks are well established by adulthood. But faculties such as movement, language, sensation and vision are not in any case confined to small cortical regions: they are distributed across networks, within which shifts in emphasis may be seen and new pathways formed in response to recent and prior experience. In this way neuroplasticity allows our brains constantly to model and remodel the world we inhabit, its representations shifting like underwater sands moulded by the ebbs and flows of life's tides.

*

To understand how plasticity occurs – how activity or information arriving from the outside world can mould the brain's pathways – it is worthwhile digging a little into what happens within its synapses. These are the connections between neurons, of which each will typically receive thousands at its dendrites (inputs) and pass on thousands at the end of its axon (outputs). Consider a boxer in the ring, preparing to take a swing at his opponent. Somewhere in his left frontal lobe he has a *Prepare Right Hook* neuron (or perhaps a circuit, but let's call it a neuron for now). When this is activated it will need to trigger a number of motor programmes in parallel: to clench his right fist, pull his right arm back at the shoulder and turn his trunk slightly. He has separate neurons to activate each of these programmes and *Prepare Right Hook* has synapses with all of them, the pathway fanning out in parallel like the branches of a tree. Focusing on his *Clench Fist* neuron, this in turn needs to fire neurons controlling several hand and wrist muscles, the cascade of activation fanning out yet further. By firing his *Prepare Right Hook* neuron the boxer causes electrical activity to ripple outwards, ultimately reaching all of the relevant muscles at the same time.

When a neuron fires, an electrical voltage spike passes rapidly out of its cell body and along its axon – the long cable-like section – until it reaches the synaptic terminals. These are bulges at the axon's far end which contain stores of a neurotransmitter chemical, and they respond to the voltage spike by releasing these stores into the small gap between the terminal and the next neuron: the connection across this gap is the synapse. The neurotransmitter is a chemical messenger for the next neuron along the pathway. It latches onto receptors on that neuron's dendrites, where it causes an immediate voltage change: if this change reaches a certain threshold then *Clench Fist* will fire, in turn discharging its own synapses with the next neurons along the pathway. The 'strength' of each synapse – whether it induces a small or large voltage change – determines how likely it is to cause the next neuron in the pathway to fire, and these strengths can be adjusted individually.

The key to neuroplasticity is that a given synapse's strength changes depending on how active it has been previously. In general, the more a given synapse is fired the stronger it gets – more neurotransmitter stored at the terminal, more receptors at the receiving end, larger effect on voltage. After a thousand training punches thrown at the heavy bag the boxer's pathway from *Prepare Right Hook* to the correct muscles is strong and ready to go. In our dense forest analogy, the thin winding track is trodden by repeated use into a wide path that is easy to traverse. From this key principle flows the ability of neural networks to learn – it allows the brain's previous activity and experience to leave its imprint in the individual strengths of innumerable synapses.

That the strength of individual synapses might be adjusted by previous activity was suggested by the Canadian psychologist Donald Hebb in the late 1940s. His mathematical modelling showed that such a mechanism might in theory allow networks of neurons to retain information, and so to learn – this is known as Hebb's postulate. Nearly twenty years later, the Norwegian navy doctor turned physiologist Terje Lomo demonstrated this directly, recording tiny voltage spikes from a specific pathway in the brains of anaesthetised rabbits. After applying a rapid burst of high-intensity stimuli any subsequent single stimulus would result in a much larger response – the synapse had become more efficient and remained stronger in the long term.

The model that Hebb proposed has another important property which makes it attractive as a way of explaining how networks of neurons might learn. This 'association' is the process by which two stimuli may become linked. Advertisers depend on associative learning. When we see pictures of George Clooney drinking a particular brand of coffee we experience the warm glow that George's crinkled smile universally provokes. It is crucial that we feel the warm glow at the same time as we see the name of the coffee. If we experience these two stimuli as a pair every time we see the advert on the side of a bus then soon they become associated: the sight of the coffee alone is enough to cause the warm glow and George's work is done. This is how Pavlov could make his conditioned dogs salivate by ringing a bell.

Hebb's postulate suggests that 'neurons which fire together wire together'. In his model timing is everything: if two neurons connected in a network are active at the same time then the synapse between them gets stronger, even if one on its own would be insufficient to make the other fire. This means that because the synapse from your *Clooney* neuron to your *Warm Glow* centre is already very strong, the fact that the *This Coffee* neuron's contribution is initially weak does not matter. Because *Warm Glow* was blazing away at the same time that *This Coffee* was weakly active, the synapse linking them will now be strengthened. Soon *This Coffee* will be strong enough to make *Warm Glow* fire all by itself. Kerching.

*

Claire had been with us for almost three months. Early therapy sessions had been difficult: she would find it hard to concentrate on what she was being asked to do and was easily distracted by anything else happening in the room. It was also quite an effort for her to be hoisted into a chair and made ready for the day, and she would become tired ten or fifteen minutes into a session. As she began to get used to her new routine she gradually built up some stamina and would engage better in what we were trying to do with her. Though still not speaking, she began to use gestures more easily to communicate. With time our speech therapist Laurel also saw some possible attempts to initiate speech. In her case notes she wrote: 'Noted increased eye widening and mouth movements in response to some questions. Eye gaze shifted to others when walking past in the day room then returned to me and maintained eye contact.'

Things seemed to pick up further once music therapy was introduced. Claire's stronger right hand sprang to life when offered instruments to play, plucking avidly at the strings of a ukulele or guitar. She sat in a small room with Becky, our endlessly patient music therapist, who played a carefully chosen tune on her guitar while Claire shook along with a set of maracas. They would fall out of phase at times but her sense of timing was pretty good and playing along brought her out in a wide smile. In the next music session Laurel and Becky observed more spontaneous facial expressions than we had previously seen in Claire and she appeared more proactive, pointing to instruments to make a choice.

Day after day and session after session Laurel tried to bring out Claire's communication, drilling her to make choices and identify objects correctly or trying to engage her mouth and tongue. In one session Laurel pointed at a photo of a friend that Claire had with her and asked who she was. There was still no audible response but she could have sworn that Claire mouthed the word 'Karen'.

One morning I walked into Claire's bay and distractedly said hello as I headed past her. I was looking for Dennis and thought he might be at this end of the ward. In one hand I was cradling an illicit coffee cup (not strictly allowed on the ward) and in the other I held a patient list. Claire looked up.

'What happened to your hair?'

I stopped dead. I tried not to gape and wiped ineffectually at the coffee I had spilt on my patient list. Claire had just spoken to me. Unprompted. As it happened I had suffered a disastrous encounter with a local barber the previous day so my hair was a bit of a sore point. As I told her the story she grinned broadly.

Had I caught up properly with the therapists then I would have known that the re-emergence of Claire's speech had been coming on over the last week or so. She had started with single words in response to questions, then, when the therapists reinforced this, she began to come out with phrases or even short sentences. Claire became really quite chatty from this point, and we got used to receiving fairly fruity comments from her. She was much more present and interactive than she had been and in parallel began to make progress with using her right hand in a more functional way.

It was now more than a year after her haemorrhage and before coming to our unit she had been static for months. There were probably some medical factors at play. Claire had arrived on high doses of anti-spasticity medication in order to counteract the extreme muscle overactivity in her legs. This is effective but also pretty sedating. We had implanted a device in her abdomen which pumped this medication directly to the base of her spinal cord, relaxing her legs and allowing us to take her off the tablets which were making her sleepy. We had also started her on a low dose of a medication to increase the availability of dopamine in her brain, with the aim of supporting the regions which promote initiation.

These medical tweaks may have helped by optimising conditions, but I have no doubt that it was neuroplasticity driven by stimulation and intensive therapy input which drove this change in her communication. The emergence of new capabilities in this way – albeit in this case an old function which had been lost – suggests to me more generally that not only is neuroplasticity still available at a late stage after stroke but it is also capable in the right environment of bringing about meaningful change.

*

Associative plasticity and the Clooney effect are all very well but our goal is not to sell coffee. If we are to learn new skills and movements – or re-learn old ones such as Claire's speech – then the adjustments in our synapses brought about by neuroplasticity must translate into changes in motor control. Learning a new skill or adapting to a change means altering the way our cortical regions relate to the outside world, much as the sensory maps shifted when Gerald Finnerty trimmed his rats' whiskers. But how can repetitive training or synaptic plasticity change the layouts of cortical maps?

The pyramidal cells of the motor cortex – the output neurons that Alexander marshalled to attack his breakfast – are all arranged heading vertically downward, but it turns out that they are also densely linked with each other by a mesh of horizontal connections sitting perpendicular to them just beneath the cortical surface. These potential connections between vertical outputs probably lie dormant for most of the time, however, actively suppressed by the inhibitory actions of small neurons which keep them in check. These cortical circuits release the neurotransmitter GABA, the brain's primary inhibitor, and by maintaining a state of inhibition effectively prevent the re-moulding of cortical maps.

The theory goes that if your cortical neurons need to access other output neurons nearby – whether in response to some change or to learn a new task – then these inhibitory circuits are somehow turned down or off. This disinhibition opens up the dormant horizontal connections, linking one output neuron to its neighbours and expanding its field of influence to surrounding regions. This might lead to an enlarged cortical map such as is seen when a monkey learns a fiddly task with its fingers, or when one of a rat's whiskers is trimmed. With training and neuroplasticity these new connections may then be strengthened.

You can bring about cortical disinhibition in healthy human subjects. Using a form of MRI scan that indirectly measures the concentration of GABA in the brain, you can detect a significant drop within the motor cortex after learning a new task involving one hand. Alternatively if you apply a tourniquet to somebody's arm and tighten it until the forearm goes numb – mimicking the sudden loss of sensory input you might see after a stroke – then you likewise see a dramatic reduction in GABA activity within the corresponding cortical regions. So not only is inhibition switched off in the cortex when learning a new task, but this also occurs within minutes when the brain suddenly loses a chunk of its input. This raises the question: could such disinhibition promote neuroplasticity and open up horizontal connections to support the recovery we see after brain injuries?

The other key ingredient for neuroplasticity is what is often called the enriched environment. If an adult rat is kept in a stimulating environment – a large cage full of activities, exercise wheels and so on – then it can correct a lazy eye by reactivating the ocular dominance plasticity usually only available in infancy. Such plasticity in response to environmental stimulation can even be visualised directly. If a mouse is given a reaching task to learn with its forearm then, using an electron microscope, you see new branches forming on the dendrites of its cortical neurons within an hour. If instead the mouse sits in a featureless cage with nothing to do then the dendrites remain static or even dwindle. When I consider this experiment I think back to Paul, the neurosurgical patient who after his brain injury was marooned in a side-room with blank walls and no therapy. I dread to think what his dendritic spines looked like.

*

I headed from the day room down the shallow ramp onto the main ward. I had a lot to do that afternoon and was trying to arrange tasks in order in my head, so I was slow to react when two young boys ran around the bend in the corridor and one careered straight into my tummy. He bounced back, recovered quickly, and looked up at me with wide eyes.

'Mummy can talk! Mummy can talk!'

He ran on past me, younger brother in tow, and they darted about the day room telling anybody who would listen. These were Claire's boys, and they had just come from her bedside. I thought I had better go and see how she was so I detoured to her bay, but far from bathing in maternal joy I found her in a foul mood. I told her I had just met her boys, and how great it was that she was now chatting to them again. She scowled.

'Pain in the fucking arse. Needs to shut up.'

This seemed a little harsh. I suggested that they were just excited to see their mum getting better – I could not blame them for being a little boisterous.

'Not my boys. Boys are great. That twat.'

Claire jabbed her right arm in the direction of the next bay along the ward. The bed nearest the corridor had the curtains pulled around it but a commotion was coming from within. This was Danny, a young lad who had been admitted a few days earlier and who had not yet settled. He was trying to climb out of his bed but was definitely too unsteady to do this by himself. Because he was intermittently confused this was a repeating pattern, so we had a member of staff sitting with him constantly. Danny was unhappy with this arrangement and was pretty vocal about it – nobody in his or Claire's bay was getting much sleep. As a result Claire had become extraordinarily grumpy and was refusing to go to therapy sessions. I realised what she was referring to.

'Ah, yes. Sorry about the noise, Claire. He isn't very well at the moment.'

She leaned forward in her wheelchair and shook her one functioning fist.

'He'll be worse in a minute if I get to him.'

I left Claire to go and find Dennis in his office. We were going to have to look at moving some beds around.

CHAPTER SIX

LEARNING TO MOVE (AGAIN)

Danny needed somebody to keep an eye on him. Left to himself he would lie placidly in his bed or sit calmly in his chair for most of the day, but every now and then a febrile restlessness would rise up within him like a sudden breeze shaking a treetop. When this happened a faraway look came into his eyes, then he looked straight through you and scrabbled about to get up on his feet. This was not a good idea, or at least not unaided: his right side was weak and his balance was all over the place. To prevent him from falling he would need either to be helped out of bed or settled back into it. His memory was sketchy when he first arrived with us, so this routine would play out several times across the day or whenever he awoke during the night. Danny's neighbours were mostly pretty understanding (unlike Claire in the next bay), but after a few nights of requests for earplugs we moved him to a side-room with a healthcare assistant to watch over him.

Danny was in his early thirties and lived in a shared house in south London. He was a tall and pale fellow, sparse of flesh, with a slight stoop and a scarecrow frame. He had gentle but nervous eyes set deeply into a gaunt face, and his complexion held a faint sheen reminiscent of raw chicken. Danny was a freelance gardener, work he loved. He took particular pleasure in building dry stone walls, carefuly laying each course in perfect alignment with a line strung between two pegs. As if to offset this quest for order within his work he liked to bet on the horses, though he was too careful ever to allow this flirtation with the forces of randomness to get him into difficulty.

Coming home one evening he let himself into the shared stairwell and started upwards. As he climbed he felt a sharp pain envelop the base of his skull and press its way inward from behind, as if a knife were being driven into the back of his neck. He felt himself stagger on the stairs and his right leg began to give way. He knew he was not going to make it to the top floor so as he reached the first-floor landing he tried to hammer on a door with his fists but found that he was unable to lift his right arm. He banged on the landing's two doors with his left hand but nobody was in and the terrible spinning feeling that had risen within him was pulling him downwards.

Danny was found unconscious on the stairwell by a neighbour a few minutes later. He had bled from a rogue blood vessel sitting within his pons, on the left side of his brainstem, and needed surgery to decompress the base of his brain. He also needed a drain to prevent the fluid in his ventricles from accumulating and this protruded from the top of his skull for a couple of weeks before being removed. As he emerged from the fog of a month on intensive care he entered a state of agitated confusion, pulling at tubes and lines and climbing out of bed to escape people he was convinced were trying to kill him. Danny needed fairly heavy-duty sedative medication in order to be managed safely but this phase gradually passed.

By the time he reached our care Danny was mainly lucid, aware most of the time where he was and what had happened, and was increasingly conscious of his physical limitations. His right arm and leg were weak. He could just about bend or straighten his arm if you supported him at the elbow but not otherwise, and he had no grip in his right hand. His left side was stronger but poorly coordinated and that arm would jerk about uncontrollably when he tried to hold something. He had double vision that came and went and he slurred his words.

We found that Danny got on better with some staff than with others, and we kept aspects of his daily routine as consistent as possible. We put up a sign by his bed which reminded him where he was and why, with the current date and a clock. As he settled into his stay with us, we were able to wean him off the anti-psychotic medication that had been started on intensive care. His side-room had been helpful while he was more restless, but this low-stimulation environment would not ultimately lead to much change. So over the first weeks we gradually got him out for therapy more and increased the time he spent in the day room.

Here he began to blossom. Having been reserved and rather shy in conversation he came out of his shell once he began to sit in groups at mealtimes. He took a shine to Claire (who had forgiven him for the noisy nights and no longer threatened to punch his lights out), detecting in her perhaps somebody who was having a harder time than he was. As soon as he was able to punt his wheelchair about with his legs he would regularly check on her at lunch, making jokes about her love of One Direction and asking a staff member to get her a cup of tea. Claire would respond with a grunt or a few gruff words, accompanied by a shrug of her right arm and, sometimes, a flash of a smile.

I went to greet them in the day room one morning but before I could say hello Claire grabbed me with her right arm. Her eyes were bright and she looked more animated than I had seen her for a while.

'The arm is moving, look. Can lift it up! Lift it up!'

For all the progress Claire was making in her communication her left arm had remained stubbornly lifeless so I thought this might be wishful thinking on her part. I was considering how to respond without squishing her excitement when she let go of me and jabbed at Danny's right arm.

'Go on, Danny, show him.'

Sure enough Danny lifted his hand off the table and brought it to his mouth. He then made half a fist and was able to open his fingers slowly back out again. Claire was right: Danny had new movement in his weak arm.

*

When a brain injury causes weakness most people, though not all, will afterwards see a degree of recovery with time. Some of this will be spontaneous and some will depend on therapy. Most neuro-trained therapists know this instinctively but it has been slow to filter its way through to either patients or doctors. To enhance or in some way unleash this natural recovery is the holy grail of rehabilitation neuroscience.

We have heard in earlier chapters how cortical maps may be fluid, their representations shifting in response to training or a change in circumstances. It has become apparent that this form of plasticity occurs also after a stroke, and may be instrumental in the recovery process. Randolph Nudo and his colleagues in Texas studied squirrel monkeys in the 1990s to examine how their control of movement changes after a stroke. They made a small hole over the motor cortex and by blocking off a blood vessel caused a stroke of around two millimetres diameter within the area controlling the hand. Unsurprisingly the monkey's hand would become weak and difficult to use, but with time normal function would gradually return. Left to its own devices the monkey's hand would recover fully over about two months. If they actively trained the weaker hand to pick up food pellets then this process would take only three or four weeks.

By mapping out the intact cortex surrounding the stroke – stimulating individual neurons and seeing which muscles they controlled – Nudo's team could see that the motor maps shifted as recovery progressed. The pattern of change they saw depended on the training the monkey underwent after the stroke. In the untrained group the weak hand's representation in this region would shrink – neurons around the stroke would instead control shoulder and upper arm muscles. In the trained group the hand's representation would be maintained or would even expand into neighbouring regions. Some monkeys, however, made good recoveries without any perceptible changes in the representations. Cortical maps, then, must only be part of the story.

After Nudo's monkey experiments it was not long before people were using magnetic stimulation to study motor maps in people with stroke and sure enough similar shifts could be seen. The representation of the weak arm would initially shrink and as recovery progressed it would re-enlarge. The late 1990s and early 2000s also saw an explosion of interest in applying the newly developed functional brain imaging techniques to this question: you perform an MRI scan while the subject carries out a specific task and by visualising changes in blood flow see which brain regions they are using. In a healthy subject making a gripping movement with their right hand you would expect them to use mainly their left motor cortex, and indeed this 'lights up' on the scan. In a patient who is recovering from a stroke, though, the pattern looks very different. When they squeeze with their weaker hand an entire network lights up, including some areas on the opposite side of the brain. These are mostly regions which are part of the normal wider motor network, but they would not usually be so active during a simple squeezing movement. So what are they doing? And why is the brain's other hemisphere getting involved?

When I first became aware of this growing field as a junior doctor the new investigative techniques were asking more questions than people had time to answer. The idea of post-stroke brain plasticity seemed like a Wild West, with cowboys all around and open frontiers in every direction. As I arrived at Queen Square to start a PhD I was lucky to have a legend for a sheriff. John Rothwell is a softly spoken and understated Lancastrian whose gentle lilt and unassuming manner give little sense of the titanic command he exerts over his field. When I arrived at his lab he was taking research fellows from all over the world, most seeking to use the magnetic stimulation technique he had developed to study the workings of the human motor cortex. Having known John for over twenty years I have not once seen him in anything other than bright red socks.

On my first day I sat in John's office and he sketched out on a piece of blank paper the outline of a planned study which would follow changes in the motor cortex of stroke patients over a period of time. As he patiently explained his idea to me I sneaked a look around his study, whose windows gave onto the treetops of the square. There were back issues of the journal *Brain*, copies of another called *Experimental Brain Research* and hard-bound copies of PhD theses he had supervised, standardised chunky blue volumes with gold lettering. There were even some of his prodigious predecessor David Marsden's books on the shelves. As I took this all in it occurred to me that I had absolutely no idea what I was doing. I could manage a ward full of ill people and had decent medical knowledge – I could probably cobble together a list of the causes of clubbing of the nails, for example – but when it came to this sort of research I was greener than Kermit, a medical interloper in a place of science. If John picked up on my nervousness he did not show it. He took me through to one of the labs, introduced me to one of his research fellows who would show me the ropes, and left me to it.

These labs became my haunt and I found it was easy to lose myself within them for hours at a time. Racks of instruments stretched up dingy walls to high ceilings. Motes of dust floated slowly across high frosted windows and cast shadows onto dark Edwardian wooden floors, creating the feel more of an apothecary than a modern lab. On the racks sat equipment that looked like it had been there for years: oscilloscopes with small round green screens, enormous amplifiers with rows of sockets and lines of cables joining them to the levels above. Wires hung from racks and pegs like red and grey foliage. On trolleys sat large magnetic stimulators, grey metal boxes attached by thick cables to insulated copper coils shaped like figures-of-eight.

We had a lab for studying balance, complete with force plates for standing on, chairs that spun round, long metal wires that connected to pulleys on the ceiling and galvanic stimulators – devices that stimulated your inner ear and induced an odd sensation of tilting to one side. I once poked my head into one of the labs to find an elderly gentleman sitting in a chair connected by several wires to the various machines, applying an electrical stimulator to his own arm while peering at an oscilloscope. I learned that he was a distinguished but retired professor who had come in to test a hunch – I left him to it.

It turned out not to be too difficult to work these gadgets and, as always in science, the key lay in knowing what question you were trying to answer. I learned that by applying John's techniques you could use these magnetic stimulators to assess not only the connection from the motor cortex to the muscles of the arm but also the activity in circuits that live within the cortex itself. The patient or healthy subject being tested (referred to by my wife as 'your victims') would sit semi-recumbent in an armchair while I attached electrodes to muscles on their hand to record the activity within them. I say armchair, but in fact the seat in the lab I used most often was a repurposed car seat whose origins were obscure.

With the subject seated I would then stand behind them and hold one of the figure-of-eight coils over their motor cortex, resting it gently on the scalp, and every few seconds the stimulator would deliver through it a short but very powerful electric pulse. None of the electricity would reach the subject but it would induce a brief and focused magnetic field just beneath the coil and within the subject's cerebral cortex. This would be strong enough to cause the axons of those neurons to discharge, triggering a volley of activity in them that would reach wherever was their target. You knew you were in the right place for the motor cortex because with each click of the stimulator the relevant body part would give a twitch – a bit like tapping a knee jerk but from the brain. Once you had located the most effective spot to move your target hand muscle you would see a big spike of electrical response on the screen. Having done this you would make a mark on the scalp with a crayon to fix the spot.

Reading it back this sounds rather amateurish, and people now use motion detection devices linked to brain scans to get a more accurate fix, but even with these simple methods you could achieve pretty reliable results. The intensity of the pulses could be adjusted by turning a large dial on the stimulator's side up or down (very *Rocky Horror Show*). By giving two pulses separated by a few milliseconds, one weak and one stronger, you could stimulate the small inhibitory neurons which sit within the cortex and this resulted in a smaller overall response – the size of this inhibitory effect would tell you how active these neurons were. In fact by varying the time interval between two pulses you could test a variety of intracortical circuits in this way.

Having spent a few months playing around with these machines and perfecting the techniques, I began to do studies with patients on the hospital's stroke ward. I managed to co-opt a cupboard to store my gear and I would drag the heavy machinery out on two large trolleys for each patient session, setting up a temporary lab in the ward's gym.

I described in the last chapter how the horizontal connections linking adjacent output cells in our motor cortex are kept suppressed by the inhibitory actions of small regulatory neurons, preventing changes in cortical organisation. This form of local inhibition can be measured directly using magnetic stimulation: studies by others had previously shown that it is reduced in many patients after stroke, not only on the affected side of the brain but also within the intact hemisphere. We replicated this finding but also found that the more severe the stroke the more this inhibition was reduced. With time as our patients recovered (to varying degrees) it tended to normalise.

We combined the magnetic stimulation technique with functional MRI scans and found that we could correlate the severity of the stroke (smaller hand responses to stimulation) with the extent to which stroke patients were accessing a wider motor network to move the weaker hand. So was it the case that turning the usual inhibition within the cortex down or off was some sort of adaptive response to the stroke? Maybe if the usual projection from our motor cortex to our hand is interrupted then switching off inhibitory circuits allows us to open up the usually dormant horizontal connections to neighbouring regions, and by doing so access alternative projections to the hand? Could we even be accessing projections to regions on the other side of the brain to support movement?

The idea that switching off inhibition outsources the job of moving the hand to other cortical regions is an attractive one, but it is probably an over-simplification. The newly involved brain regions may be active during hand movement after stroke but it is far from clear what they are doing and whether they are being helpful. In fact, there is a school of thought that the activity we see in the non-stroke hemisphere may even be getting in the way. When Alexander in Chapter 4 was using both hands to cut his cylindrical pork-based breakfast item (I made a promise) his motor cortices on either side were talking to each other via the corpus callosum. You can test that interaction in healthy people using two magnetic coils – one on each side of the head – and, when we are not moving, the two sides inhibit each other. When we are about to make a hand movement this inhibition is usually switched off, but an influential study in patients with stroke showed that for them it remained active as they tried to move their weak hand. This was interpreted as suggesting that an over-active non-stroke hemisphere – released from the other side's usual inhibitory influence – was somehow now interfering with the stroke hemisphere's attempts to make normal movements, its own inhibition spilling over and getting in the way.

This concept has been called the interhemispheric imbalance model and it gave rise to a large number of attempts to rebalance brain activity after stroke, artificially 'turning down' what was seen as a pathologically overactive non-stroke motor cortex in order to improve the recovery of movement. You can do this using either a series of magnetic pulses or a small electrical current applied over the scalp for a few minutes, causing an excitability change that can outlast the stimulation by an hour or more. So, if you can adjust the activity in specific brain regions for periods of time then perhaps you could eliminate the pesky inhibition coming from the non-stroke side during therapy and so produce better recovery outcomes.

There have been many studies like this, some increasing activity on the stroke side and others reducing it on the non-stroke side, almost all with small patient numbers. Some showed a beneficial effect on recovery while others did not, and for all the excitement that this approach has generated the consensus now is that there is either little effect or it is not reliable enough to be clinically useful. So brain stimulation for hand weakness has not found its way into clinical practice, though you will still find its devotees.

It should perhaps not be that surprising that a tool as blunt as magnetic or electrical stimulation does not somehow unleash better stroke recovery. Magnetic stimulation affects an area around the size of a coin while electrical stimulation is felt across most of one hemisphere, which means these interventions are having a blanket effect across billions of neurons. To me this seems like banging the top of a faulty television – you don't really know what you are doing but it often seems to have some sort of effect. New stimulation techniques are being developed now that are more focused and more sophisticated in how they align with the brain's electrical rhythms, so it is still possible that this approach may bear fruit.

*

The nights were drawing in, the long windows were dark by teatime and sparkly reindeer were beginning to appear around the day room. The therapists were planning the Christmas quiz and had given in to Claire's insistence on including a 2010s boyband round. Danny was making great progress across the board. To get out of bed and into a chair he had needed two people to help him but he was now doing this on his own. The therapists had given him an actual script for this process – roll onto my side, swing my legs over the edge, push up and hold on, reach out and hold the frame, etc. – and he recited this out loud as he completed each step in order to counteract his tendency to charge ahead. With time and practice he began to manage without the script.

Soon Danny could take steps with support from the physios and gradually he moved on to walking with a Nordic pole, a kind of long stick. His left arm would still wobble and jerk about, and the right was not yet strong enough to be useful, but the pole acted as a steadying influence. In a similar vein the therapists gave him wrist weights for his left arm and he began to be able to use the microwave to heat up food. The nurses gradually involved themselves less in his daily routine of washing and dressing and we started 'independence days', where they would leave him to his own devices and then check in with him later on. Gradually his confidence grew.

I found myself in the brain injury education group with four patients including Danny and Claire. In broad terms I talked them through the normal functions of the various brain regions, holding tightly onto the pin that held the plastic model together in a vain effort to prevent its usual collapse. We were all trying politely to ignore the fact that Stewart had nodded off in his wheelchair. Danny sat forward and asked occasional questions while Claire, who appeared to be taking it all in, looked on in inscrutable silence.

I got to the part about stroke, explaining what it is and the different sorts of difficulties it can cause depending on the brain regions affected. I told them that the damaged area does not grow back, but that the surviving brain tissue is good at re-organising and forming new connections. This is driven by therapy and practice and can lead to a degree of recovery. As if to illustrate my point Danny lifted his weaker right arm off his lap and plomped it onto the table with a thud (Stewart snorted briefly but went back to sleep). Claire looked up at me and nodded towards her left side which was still showing no signs of life.

'So why isn't my arm moving?'

I explained that depending on the site and extent of the damage people tend to change at different rates. Sometimes a limb will remain weak despite all the therapy we can give it, but when that happens we can usually still find ways to improve somebody's independence. She raised her eyebrows and looked away with a weary shrug.

'Bad luck, I guess,' she muttered. 'Always the same. Bad luck, Claire.'

*

Often following a stroke which causes complete weakness down one side – so-called hemiplegia – you will start to see some movement in the leg within a week or so while the arm remains inert. This has nothing to do with reorganisation or plasticity and simply reflects the anatomical fact that the tracts to the leg are quite often not directly damaged. They are compromised by swelling and inflammation in the nearby damaged brain – as this all settles down those tracts wake up again and the leg moves. The affected arm, assuming it improves, will then typically follow a fairly stereotyped sequence of steps over the coming month or so. These stages were first noted in monkeys by Sir Charles Sherrington (coiner of the word 'synapse'), who caused experimental damage to their motor cortex and then noted a sequence of spontaneous recovery towards normal use of the arm. This was fleshed out in greater detail for humans by American neurologist Thomas Twitchell and then by physiotherapist Signe Brunnström. After an initial period of complete flaccid weakness patients will typically first develop some flexion (bending movement) at the shoulder, then also at the elbow and then the wrist and fingers, but only as part of a synergy – the joints cannot be moved separately and can only flex together. A while later some extension (straightening movement) will appear, starting at the shoulder and working its way down, but again only as part of a synergy. The patient will then gradually develop both flexion and extension movements in individual joints without synergy, and eventually individual finger and thumb movements, leading ultimately to full functional use of the arm.

This sequence considers only weakness but in practice a number of other factors may also get in the way: muscle stiffness, pain, loss of sensation, cognitive difficulties with movement. This also presumes a full recovery, while in practice a patient's progress may well stall along the way. Like Claire's. Alternatively if somebody is not lucky enough to encounter a good therapist during this process they may learn unhelpful compensatory movements as recovery progresses. Clearly, though, there is a biological process going on, presumably in the surviving brain tissue, that is allowing these changes to occur. In fact we now know that there is an awful lot going on at the cellular level, much of which has been learned from animal models.

At the core of a stroke is brain tissue which has lost its blood supply and has died. As the cells perish they break down and lose their structure, becoming jellied gloop. As in other tissues such as skin, surrounding cells react to cell death by forming scar tissue – in the brain this is called gliosis – and a thin fibrous wall forms around the stroke's core. Immediately around this is tissue which suffered a reduced blood supply but has just about survived, known as the peri-infarct zone. This injured tissue reacts by releasing chemical messengers called cytokines which attract and switch on a host of inflammatory cells. These in turn release damaging chemicals called free radicals (the kind which expensive shampoos love to mop up, the better to protect your hair) and more cytokines. These leach out into the surrounding brain tissue where, for days or even weeks, they have a profound activating effect on all cell types: not just the neurons themselves but also the supporting cells (astrocytes) and blood vessels.

All this means that the cells in the brain tissue around the stroke find themselves in a chemical environment that irritates and activates them. In the neurons this triggers growth programmes, switching on genes that were last active when the brain was developing: as a result their dendrites start to form new branches and their axons begin to grow and sprout, leading to new synaptic connections between these surviving neurons and neighbouring regions. This provides fertile ground for new pathways to form and is probably responsible for much of the early spontaneous recovery we see – if you block axonal sprouting then you block recovery. If the newly forming synapses can be trained with therapy into functioning neural pathways then we may begin to see the re-emergence of lost functions – in this case movement.

*

Danny's right arm continued to improve and when the rehab assistants took our Connect 4 set out of its box in the day room he began to show some interest in giving it a go. It was hard at first but with their encouragement he soon experimented with using his right hand to hold the counters instead of his stronger but jerkier left side. We like Connect 4 in rehab – it is an excellent therapeutic upper limb task with additional cognitive elements. The more Danny played, the easier it gradually became for him to get his hand up to the top of each column. The hardest part for him was to open up his hand to release the counters but once he had mastered this he began to mind where the counters were falling and who was winning – the game was on.

Rather to our surprise Claire could also manage this with her right arm and once her two young boys realised this they would run and get the box each time they arrived for a visit, the younger one climbing up on a chair to reach the top shelf. They excitedly set up the game on one of the tables, arranging the two sets of counters in neat stacks before her, and sat playing it for long periods. They patiently steered their mother's hand to the top of the tray until they were confident she could manage it. At first her boys had to remind Claire of the rules but in fact she turned out to be pretty good – despite her ongoing cognitive difficulties her Connect 4 circuits seemed bizarrely to have been spared. When one of her counters dropped to the bottom of its slot and made a row of four her boys whooped with delight. She confined herself to a gruff harrumph.

Claire began to take Danny on in a regular game at lunchtime. As I passed one day he sat across from her wheelchair at one of the tables while her boys looked eagerly on like spectators at a high-stakes poker table. The game was slow and although Claire's boys egged her on, peering and leaning in with each move she made, they sat on their hands to avoid actually helping her. From a table nearer the coffee machine I could see Jeremy watching on discreetly. An athletic man of around sixty with tightly combed wavy hair and glasses, he reminded me of a grey Clark Kent. Jeremy had run his own small business pretty successfully until a bike accident had landed him on ICU with a brain injury. He had a number of resulting difficulties and although these were changing, progress was slow: it was beginning to look like he would still need some help when he went home.

Jeremy's wife Lauren was much younger than him, salon-fresh blonde hair always immaculate, and tight-lipped with the stress of the situation she found herself in. She had married a thrusting entrepreneur with prospects – disability was not in the script. She pushed Jeremy harder and harder with each visit, demanding longer therapy sessions and drilling him with exercises well into the evening, until the therapists had to explain that he also needed to rest. Jeremy bore up under this additional pressure but a few days earlier had broken down and confessed to his physio that Lauren had threatened to leave him if he did not recover. Watching the Connect 4 game play out across the day room Jeremy's eyes brightened and he looked like he wanted to join in, but Lauren was trying to put his weak hand around a glass so he turned back to her.

Claire completed her row and Danny's broomstick-like frame shook as he looked up at me from hooded eyes and laughed.

'She's too good for me!'

Claire gave an eye roll and a modest shrug but I could see she was suppressing a smile.

This was the usual pattern: Claire mostly won these lunchtime duels with Danny. Though I could not be sure he was not going a little easy on her.

*

The activation of neuronal growth processes after a stroke is not limited to the region just around the damage. The neurons of the motor cortex have long axons which reach distant regions, projecting down to the spinal cord and across the midline to their counterparts in the opposite hemisphere. When these neurons are involved in a stroke these long axons slowly degenerate and as they do so this triggers activation of cellular growth programmes in these remote regions similar to that seen at the site of damage. In rats with stroke you will begin to see axonal sprouting in motor regions on the other side of the brain, in time even forming new projections from that side down to the brainstem and the spinal cord. Crucially, the extent of axonal sprouting seen in this animal model is much greater if they are engaged in learning a new task: something about this activated post-stroke state enhances the neurons' response to the stimulation of training.

The question of what exactly the overactive regions of the non-stroke hemisphere are doing during attempts to move is still not fully answered. While there is some evidence in humans that they may be impeding the recovering arm, the jury really is out on this: suppressing these regions during stroke recovery has not produced consistent benefits and in more severely affected patients can even make the movement worse. In Sherrington's monkeys, whose arms had recovered very well following damage to their motor cortex, a second procedure damaging the cortex on the opposite side did not cause the previous weakness to re-emerge. A similar experiment in rats, however, found that the second procedure undid recovery of forelimb movement in the more severely affected animals, but only if new projections down to the brainstem were targeted. So if we can extrapolate this to human stroke – and that's a big if – it may be that in patients with more limited recovery the non-stroke hemisphere is to some extent propping up residual movement using a rather slow and roundabout new route to the arm via the brainstem.

*

Claire's recovery had hit a plateau and we had reached the limit of what we could usefully change in the inpatient setting. While Danny's right arm seemed to gain new capabilities with each passing week – he had started cooking now, using both hands together – Claire's left side remained stubbornly lifeless, as did her right leg. By this point it was clear that she was not going to regain movement in those limbs and she understood this. She had much better use of her right arm than previously, and her speech continued to become more spontaneous, but with three non-functional limbs out of four plus a fair amount of cognitive difficulty Claire was always going to need some looking after.

The flat she shared with her partner and their boys was too small to accommodate the hoist she would need to get in and out of bed and her wheelchair would not fit into their bathroom. Getting her into the flat in the first place would also only be possible if she were physically lifted in by a four-man crew. Discharging her there was not really feasible. Claire and her partner rented their flat from the local council and had already requested rehousing – our social worker had made sure that they were in the top priority bracket – but even for somebody in Claire's situation councils often take well over a year to find somewhere suitable. So after much discussion it was decided that when she left us Claire would move to a care home. Once her family were rehoused they would look at setting things up so that she could move back in with them. Claire was initially against this plan, as almost anyone would be when faced with the idea of not living at home, but on the basis that it was hoped to be temporary she grudgingly came round.

Looking in on Claire, I asked her how she was feeling about leaving us. She was sitting out in her wheelchair and when I came in had been watching something on a tablet propped up on her bedside table. This was piled up with magazines and cards from her family, and I wheeled it to one side so that I could perch on her bed. The tall blue pleated curtain was pulled around us and the harsh lights beamed down from above.

'Well, I can't stay in hospital for ever, can I? Got to get on. Got to get on.'

I pointed out that one of the positives of the care home would be that it would be easy for her to get in and out. As well as her family visiting her there she could meet them outside and go on trips if she wanted. She gave me a look and was silent for a while.

'Not the same though, is it?'

I couldn't disagree. It wasn't the same.

*

The biological processes that support return of movement are working at full tilt during the early post-stroke period – the question is to what extent will recovery progress? A measure of arm function at thirty days predicts longer-term recovery pretty accurately. For patients with mild or moderate impairment you can make a reasonable prediction of eventual recovery based on their arm function as early as three days post-stroke. According to a landmark study by John Krakauer and colleagues these patients will recover approximately 70 per cent of their lost function from this point to three months in what is now known as the Proportional Recovery Rule. But for patients whose early weakness is severe the situation seems to be less predictable.

Around half of these will improve as predicted by this rule but the other half will show little or no change.

These non-recoverers seem to be the patients who have no remaining projection from their cortex to their arm, and it makes intuitive sense that with this gone no amount of reorganisation in the cortex is going to make a difference. You can to some extent identify this subgroup by assessing the projection using magnetic stimulation or MRI scanning. In those with severe early weakness but an intact projection the recovery that we do see tends to start later and to take place more slowly – presumably because more extensive reorganisation must first take place for new connections to access descending pathways and so move the arm.

So if recovery over the first months is fairly predictable what is it, then, that therapy is actually doing in this early period? We know from animal models that early training enhances axonal sprouting, and from Nudo's monkeys that it speeds up recovery. Clinical experience would also suggest that therapy is needed to foster and optimise the conditions that will allow natural recovery to progress. This may involve, for example, treating any developing stiffness as it emerges, keeping the muscles and joints in good condition (and pain free), avoiding despondency and preventing the patient picking up and learning abnormal movement patterns.

This last point is crucial: there is good evidence that favouring the return of more normal movements over compensatory patterns affects the eventual usefulness of the arm. A group from Japan studied macaques with weak arms following stroke, monitoring their ability to use precision grip movements to get food pellets out of small holes. If they were trained intensively in the task starting within a few days then they recovered full function by one or two months. Without any training they still regained movement but they could not use it precisely enough to perform the fiddly task: they tended instead to make abnormal compensatory movements which were less effective. But here is the key observation: around a month after the stroke both groups started making some precision grip movements but in the untrained group they soon disappeared again. Instead of becoming locked in to their movement repertoire these new movements were lost in favour of easier but ultimately less precise compensatory movements. This is a nice illustration of how spontaneous recovery and training might interact, ensuring that emerging movements are correctly used and that the most effective patterns become embedded.

We know, then, that there is something different about the brain's biology in this early period after stroke, at least in animal models, which allows for a fruitful interaction between spontaneous recovery and training. This has given rise to the concept of a critical period – or a 'plasticity window' – during which the response to therapy is greatest. There is direct evidence for this in mice, whose forelimbs recover fully from experimental stroke if they are trained within two days but not if trained later, and some recent signs of a similar period in humans.

The idea that early therapy is important after stroke does seem to have entered mainstream consciousness. Patients or relatives will often express impatience to move onto the rehabilitation unit in order to get going, and sometimes they have read or been told that all recovery will stop at three months. This should not be over-interpreted. Every patient's clinical course is different. If somebody has a particularly severe stroke and has been drowsy or unwell for many weeks then the best time for their intensive rehab will be when they are ready and able to benefit from it, critical period or not. There is also a particular danger in the idea of a plasticity window somehow slamming shut at three months. This is sometimes used by policy makers to justify a lack of therapy input at later time points, on the basis that further change is not possible. Anybody who works in neurorehabilitation knows that for many people this is simply incorrect. True, a patient like Claire who had a stroke six or more months ago and still has no arm movement at all is unlikely to regain it. But if there is some residual movement then we know that it is often possible to improve it with intensive therapy input even a year or more down the line.

Colleagues at my hospital – Kate Kelly, Fran Brander and Nick Ward – carried out a seminal study in 2018. They treated over two hundred patients with weak arms after stroke in an intensive programme of arm therapy – ninety hours over three exhausting weeks. All patients had some movement already but were struggling to use their arm in daily tasks. The therapy was tailored to individual needs, a combination of occupational therapy and physio aiming to improve movement patterns in tasks that were meaningful for them. At the end of three weeks, impairment scores had improved on average by over 25 per cent. Tested again at six weeks and then at six months, the improvements were sustained or even slightly better. The patients had begun to incorporate their stroke arm more into daily life so they were now effectively doing their own therapy at home. But here is the kicker: these patients were on average eighteen months down the line from their stroke. All the spontaneous post-stroke biological changes would have plateaued long before then, and they would be well out of what anyone would consider a critical window of plasticity. And yet even at that late time point skilled therapy could still bring about meaningful change.

You can argue about what such a late change means. We know that these patients were not just making compensatory movements – the quality of their movements had improved, as had their efficiency. It is possible that strengthening effects play a role in unmasking existing movements, which you would not strictly call learning. But to me it is not so surprising that this result is possible. We all have the capacity to learn new movements and we do so every day. When we get a new PIN number or learn a new piece on the piano we are engaging the neuroplasticity mechanisms needed to encode these new movements – dendritic branching, changes in synapses and so on. There is no reason that I can see why a stroke patient in the chronic period, assuming they have a degree of movement and some functioning motor cortex, cannot access such mechanisms in the same way. Other studies have replicated the principle that such late change is possible and together they give the lie to the pessimistic viewpoint that has become all too prevalent.

*

Claire had got used to the idea that she would be moving to a care home and as her discharge from hospital approached she even began to get excited about it. Chatting to her at the bedside I suggested that now her right arm was so much better she could maybe make her boys something for when they visited. I reminded her that in a session in our kitchen she had already made brownies.

'Brownies, brownies.' Claire still displayed echolalia, often repeating the last thing you had said to her, apparently without noticing she was doing it. I asked what she would most like to cook for them. A grin played on her lively features.

'A parrot. I'd like to cook a parrot.'

We both laughed. Claire's plan to cook a parrot was a running joke. We had no idea where it had come from but her partner told us that she would equally have made off-beat jokes before the stroke – this was nothing new. As she talked her right hand scratched away at her chin. This had developed as a habit: when she was not engaged in something purposeful her active right arm would often worry away at something, another example of perseveration. We had ended up finding a soft glove for her to wear on her right hand to prevent skin abrasions. Being Claire she had had this glove pimped in Michael Jackson style.

When the great day for Claire's departure finally came the therapists, nurses and everyone who was around gathered at the door of the day room and we all clapped her out. Danny stood in line with the team as we waved her off. He had just presented her with a cake he had made in his occupational therapy session. On its top in green and red coloured icing was a drawing: a parrot.

We watched as the transport crew pushed Claire's chair out of the unit and down the corridor. The back of her head receded slowly from view and I could see her right arm bobbing up and down as she went. Whether she was scratching at something or waving goodbye I could not tell.

CHAPTER SEVEN

UNABLE TO ACCESS SERVER

That morning was much like any other London day in early March. The pallid air still held a cold edge and there was as yet no hint of spring. The grey lid of a sky sat limply over the city and suffused it with a feeble light.

Vikas was in a bad way and had been for some time. He worked part-time as a roofer and had joined a new job that morning, but he had a terrible hangover and the previous night was a blur. Left to himself at the front of the site a wave of nausea came over him and he found himself clinging onto a gable, looking down on the scurrying masses from three storeys above and thinking that he really should have called in sick. Nobody asked him what he was doing there or checked if he was OK, the city's bustle providing but a fragile illusion of community. In the street's buffeting stream, everyone was in their own bubble.

Vikas's foot caught in the guttering and, as he stepped back, he tried to catch the gable's edge. One moment he was on the roof and the next he was not. As a crumpled heap on the pavement he stopped the street's flow and broke its spell. Headphones came off and phones were brought out. Having stopped in their tracks a group stood about in amazed horror and remembered if only for a few minutes, as they rushed to help, that together they were part of the same great enterprise.

The ambulance took Vikas a little further than usual in order to reach a Major Trauma Centre, a hospital that would be able to handle his obviously severe injuries. The paramedics had found him to be deeply unconscious despite their efforts to rouse him, his pupils dilated and unresponsive to the lights they flashed in his eyes. He was breathing and had a pulse, but apart from the fractured limbs there was also a bloodied wound on the left side of his head and signs of damage to his chest wall with a collapsed lung. The paramedics had put a hard collar around his neck and a breathing tube down into his trachea before moving him. Now they flew through the streets in a wailing tornado of flashing light of which the passing crowds were once again only vaguely aware.

On arrival at hospital Vikas underwent a 'trauma series' of CT scans and X-rays covering all areas of evident or potential injury. Long bones were broken in both arms and in his left leg (where his shattered femur was sticking out through the skin) and one lung was indeed collapsed, needing a drain to be inserted. There were fractures of facial bones and broken teeth. He remained unconscious and this was not surprising: the scan showed skull fractures and a collection of blood over his left frontal lobe pushing the whole brain over to the right. The neurosurgeons removed a section of bone to relieve the pressure, leaving a skull defect. The orthopaedic surgeons picked off dirty and damaged tissue around the elbows and in the left leg, leaving an external fixation device to keep the thigh bone in place. Over the first week Vikas went to theatre most days for orthopaedic or neurosurgical procedures, after which he had a tracheostomy tube in his neck, a drain sticking out of his skull and an intracranial bolt to measure the pressure. By the end of the first month his theatre reward card had nine stamps on it.

Vikas was slow to wake up and, at this stage, was still not opening his eyes or trying to communicate. As well as the collection around the brain's edge his CT scan had also showed bruising within both frontal lobes and flecks of blood further down towards the centre. There was also blood around the brainstem, with possible damage to the nerve from his left eye. Slowly around this time he began to rouse, opening his eyes to sound and making eye contact with nurses. One day he opened his eyes and, turning to his right, caught sight of his mother sitting silently in the chair next to his hospital bed. Vikas reached out to her and tried to sit forward, pulling himself up in a jolt on the plastic rails of the cot sides. But he could not get enough purchase and was having to work against the air mattress, so he sank back again. She took his hand through the rails and held it.

'It's all right, love, I'm here. You just rest.'

By six weeks Vikas was more awake and starting to communicate. His left arm was stuck in a semi-flexed position with only a few degrees of available movement due to the severity of his elbow injury. The joints in his legs were mostly OK after all the surgery except for his left knee, which would not bend more than a little. He returned for yet another operation – this time to chisel off some new bone which had grown around the knee since his injury – and then the joint was able to bend. Soon after this the team removed the tracheostomy from his neck and could sit him out of bed for short periods in a tilting chair.

Now that Vikas was awake for some of the time and could speak, it became apparent that he was profoundly confused. He was mixing up words, which did not help ('Nurse, I have a pain in my ark, no, my armour . . . my arm is splurting'), but he was also unable to hold onto information for more than a few minutes so was disorientated for much of the time. Staff would remind him where he was and why, and he could then repeat this back to them, but if asked again five minutes later he would have no idea what they had said. In these periods he would at times get worked up and try to climb out of bed to get to work.

'I have to get to the fright . . . the site. The gaffer will get the hump. Why are you stopping me?'

He needed watching at all hours to keep him safe during this phase, which went on for over a month. As his memory gradually stirred into action he became more settled and he began to take part in some of the activities which the therapists were encouraging him to try – simple things at first, like sitting up and brushing his teeth. They noticed that his memory was somewhat selective, more reliable for football results than for staff members' names. In between relevant conversation he would still talk nonsense for minutes at a time, jumping rapidly between topics, and he was easily distracted by any goings-on around him.

By two months or so Vikas had undergone pretty much all of the surgery he would need and seemed at least to be stable, though clearly very impaired. At some point in the next six months the skull defect would need fixing but otherwise his medical needs were reducing and the focus began to move towards neurorehabilitation. We got the call.

*

Head injuries are unbelievably common. Each year in the UK there are around 200,000 which are serious enough to need hospital admission. Here, as in the US, many are the result of falls in the elderly or assaults in younger people, with relatively few road accidents. Those in the younger group tend to be male and there is an association with risk-taking behaviour and alcohol – men in their twenties, drinking, driving fast and getting into fights. Too often, though, the injured person was just in the wrong place at the wrong time, on a bike or crossing a road. In lower-income countries head injury is even more common – typically in the context of car accidents – and once these are included the numbers are staggering. In total each year there are around sixty million head injuries worldwide. This is largely an active and economically productive group of people and the cost has been estimated at $400 billion each year – half a per cent of the entire global output. Even those with supposedly mild brain injuries may have their lives derailed by the effects, which are very often not picked up by medical systems as they exist currently. This 'invisible disability' group present an enormous unmet need and are largely let down by existing services.

When somebody is hit hard on the head their brain receives a jolt, like a blancmange inside a tight jar. The skull is a sealed and unforgiving cavity, with no crumple zone. There are effectively two phases of impact: an initial acceleration on the side where the blow lands, and then a deceleration as the brain slams against the skull on the opposite side. This is called a contrecoup injury and if someone falls onto the back of their head you will typically see injuries to both frontal lobes. If you are hit by a car either as a pedestrian or a cyclist (who often 'bullseye' the windscreen), there may also be a second impact as you land.

The result is an immediate loss of consciousness. After a minor knock this may be brief, with just a few minutes of feeling dazed: the stars or birds flying around in a circle beloved of comic books. After a more significant injury, it may take much longer to come to, and the duration of unconsciousness is one marker of severity. Once the injured person gets to hospital, they will invariably have their head scanned if they are not fully awake. Skull fractures are common in this situation, but unless the bone fragments appear sunken or unstable they are usually left alone.

The principal reason to scan is to look for blood in or around the brain. Bleeding under the skull, from an artery or more commonly a vein, may press down on the brain's surface and push it over to the opposite side, as in Vikas's case. After higher velocity injuries you may also see bruising, or contusion, within the brain substance itself. If we trip and land hard on an arm or leg, apart from a bruise on the skin we also see and feel painful lumps in the underlying muscle: pockets of blood that have formed what my mother used to call an egg. The equivalent bruising in the brain appears on a scan as a speckled appearance of blood in the tissue, sometimes including a sizeable clot.

If a collection of blood is large enough to cause significant pressure or displacement then a neurosurgeon may need to remove it. The judgement as to when or if to intervene surgically may be finely balanced, as there are many circumstances in which an operation may not help or may make things worse. Often the initial plan is to watch and wait.

The principal bogeyman in this situation is raised pressure inside the skull and we now recognise that even a modest increase over a prolonged period probably has a detrimental effect on outcomes. Intracranial pressure is hard to monitor indirectly, so often a neurosurgeon will insert a pressure monitoring bolt to keep tabs on it: a device literally screwed through a small hole in the skull.

Typically, once the injured person awakes (which is gradual, not sudden as in the movies) there will be a period of confusion during which they are unable to retain any information and will be disorientated: a phase we call post-traumatic amnesia. When the brain cannot access recent memories it tends to make things up to fill in the gaps. The injured person may be able to answer biographical questions about themselves but they will often produce a stream of chat that bears no relation to reality: what they have been doing earlier that day, or how they need to get to the airport for a flight. Often there is a restless flavour to this 'confabulation', as it is called. They may try to climb out of bed, pull at tubes and generally pose a risk to themselves, as Danny had done. This is best managed by maintaining a low-stimulation environment and by gentle reassurance, but sedative medication may be needed for a while.

Why post-traumatic amnesia is seen so often is not entirely clear. The white matter tracts which connect the brain's regions over long distances bear much of the brunt of traumatic injury. In post-traumatic amnesia there is probably a disconnection between the memory centres of the hippocampus and the brain's 'default mode network', a collection of regions which are active when our brains are just ticking over and we are thinking about nothing in particular. Each cortical region may in itself be working fine, including the hippocampus, but they cannot talk to each other so the patient cannot lay down or access any new memories. As these connections begin to wake up so the short-term memory comes back online.

*

By the time Vikas arrived on our ward there was no longer any sign of agitation and we found him to be calm and agreeable. The registrar, Uroosa, had admitted him and in the following day's multi-disciplinary meeting she relayed the history and the results of her examination.

Vikas had little vision in his left eye, she told us – he could perceive a flash of light from a torch but could not count fingers or make out colours or shapes. His right eye was fine. There was subtle weakness on the right side of his face but otherwise the cranial nerves were fine and his speech was clear. He could follow a simple instruction, but if you asked him to perform an action with three steps then this would break down. His left elbow was stuck in semi-flexion, about thirty degrees off straight. The power in his arms seemed normal, however, and while his right leg was slightly weak the left was strong. The nurses were using a sliding board to get him in and out of bed and he was unsteady on his feet. His left knee was a few degrees off straight but essentially fine. His coordination was slightly impaired on the right. Uroosa had not done a formal cognitive screen, but he periodically needed to be reminded what he was doing on our unit. The nurse with us today was Joyce. She told us that the ward had had no issues with Vikas so far other than the occasional toileting mishap. She described him as 'a very polite gentleman'.

Uroosa and I went to find Vikas at his bedside. We walked past Bay 4 which was still boarded up for building works – we were assured that work was ongoing but nobody had heard any sounds from within for weeks – and found him in the next bay along. He was sitting calmly in the armchair next to his bed, his left arm bent awkwardly across his front and holding a well-thumbed paperback of Elizabeth David's classic *French Country Cooking*. He was not looking at his book, but was gazing out of the window at the treetops in the square. I imagined his default mode network humming away gently. When Uroosa called his name he gave a little start, looked up at us and smiled. He was wearing pale green hospital pyjamas, which hung a little off his delicate frame, and had the air of a man in a waiting room who was not entirely sure why he was there. He looked a decade or so older than his thirty years and I had the impression that life so far had been complicated.

Uroosa introduced us. Vikas did not remember having met her the previous day but he was polite and seemed happy to talk. He had a wispy black beard over hollow cheeks and a long ridge was visible at the left end of his hairline where the neurosurgeons had repaired his skull. I asked him what he was reading. He was initially nonplussed and when I indicated the book in his hand he seemed a little surprised to find it there. He hesitated as if uncertain whether to confide in us then gave a slightly embarrassed smile.

'I want to be a crook – no!' He knew this was wrong and we both laughed. 'I mean cooking. You know, a chat. No – a chef!'

This was new information, but then we had only just met.

'I thought you worked in roofing,' I volunteered.

'Well, I do. Got to pay the bills. Going to re-chain.'

I said that his plan sounded exciting and we talked a little about French dishes. He warmed to this topic and for a while was quite animated, not bothered by (or perhaps not noticing) the occasional wrong word along the way.

As a boy Vikas had visited Marseille with his mother and for dinner one evening he had been served bouillabaisse, the delicious spicy fish soup of that region. He described how the waiter had brought the rich brown broth to their table in a tall steaming bowl and had then given him a separate bowl with chunks of every fish he could imagine. This blew his ten-year-old mind and he had been perfecting his recipe ever since. His intention, once he recovered, was to serve the best bouillabaisse in London.

After a pause I asked Vikas if he knew where he was. He looked uncertain again.

'In . . . a school? Or in rehab?'

I said that was right, but then it emerged that he had meant alcohol rehab, something with which he had had a brush in the past. I told him that he was in hospital because he had been injured in a fall. Vikas looked annoyed with himself, as if he had known this all along. He had injuries to his limbs but also to his brain, I explained, which was why it was hard to remember some things at the moment. He was improving though, and was here for intensive rehab to get him back to being more independent. I asked him if he was aware of anything in his body that was not working properly. He told me everything was working fine. When we examined him he was surprised to find that he could not see out of his left eye and that his left arm would not bend.

Later that day our occupational therapist Libby took Vikas in a wheelchair to one of the interview rooms and explored how well he understood his difficulties. Was he any different now when compared to before the accident? Vikas told her he was better. Better how? He was happier. Had there been any physical changes? Yes, he was a bit different – his balance and his left arm – but he was trying to get it all back. She asked about his vision – had this changed? He said his vision was perfect. She reminded him about his left eye. He said he knew about this issue but it had been there before the accident. This was not true, but it was how he was making sense of it at that moment. How was his memory? It was good. Any problems with concentration? No, it was just the same as beforehand. Had his way of communicating changed at all? It was better – previously he was quite shy but now he was more confident in socialising. Did he have any worries about living on his own or managing daily tasks? No, he could live independently perfectly well but he did not want to just now. How about managing his finances? Someone else could deal with that. Did he have any thoughts at this stage about returning to work? He certainly planned to do this and was going to re-train as a chef, he confirmed. What was he hoping to achieve over the next six months? Happiness.

The majority of people with a traumatic brain injury – particularly those who have emerged from post-traumatic amnesia – show reduced awareness of their own impairments. 'Anosognosia' translates literally as lack of knowledge of the disease (much of the impression that doctors give of knowing what they are talking about comes simply from describing something in Ancient Greek, a sort of classical *Catchphrase* – 'Say what you see!'). This term was first coined by the French-Polish neurologist Joseph Babinski, who used it to describe two patients with right-sided stroke who flatly refused to acknowledge that they had no movement on the left side of their bodies. In traumatic brain injury the lack of insight often persists and may be present long after the patient leaves hospital.

This mismatch of perceptions can lead to fractious interactions with family members or care-givers. It also leads the patient into potentially dangerous situations – they may over-estimate their safety awareness when crossing a road, for example – and into trouble when trying to get back to work. This form of self-awareness, the ability to monitor our own performance, is sometimes called meta-cognition.

Therapists will spend much time trying to build a patient's insight into what is difficult for them and why. They may ask them to self-rate how hard they expect a task to be beforehand and then repeat the exercise afterwards. They may use group education work to build their understanding of the brain injury. They may video the patient doing the task and then watch it back with them ('I had no idea I was leaning all the way over to the left!'). Other patients may be vaguely aware that something is wrong but not bothered by it, so-called anosodiaphoria (medical *Catchphrase* again).

Much of the cognitive impairment typically seen after a traumatic brain injury can be put down to disruption of the white matter tracts that join our many cortical regions. On a special MRI sequence that images these tracts they should look like a straight bundle of dried spaghetti just before it goes into the pan – after a severe injury these tracts instead resemble the cooked article. In some ways, then, traumatic brain injury is a disease of disconnection, a failure of information flow between brain regions. This causes difficulties which can persist for years and may be hard to detect in a patient who, according to a standard medical examination, is completely intact.

Existing ways of categorising a head injury as mild, moderate or severe are extremely crude, based on clinical factors such as level of consciousness or duration of post-traumatic amnesia. These criteria probably miss a great deal of significant pathology, and now that we have more sophisticated ways of detecting damage they are due for an overhaul. As things stand, around 90 per cent of those seen in hospital with a head injury are defined as 'mild', with a normal CT scan and little or no drop in conscious level. However, around a third of these actually have small beads of haemorrhage in deep brain regions known as 'diffuse axonal injury', which can be picked up on a standard MRI scan around three weeks later. If you include sequences to look at the white matter tracts this number goes up further. But the cognitive changes are very often missed while somebody is in hospital: as long as they can walk, talk and are not obviously disorientated, people will very often be sent home.

These 'walking wounded' may have significant difficulties with their cognition, usually missed in the quick standard screens. I often see this group of patients in my clinic some months down the line at a point when they are running into difficulty. Memory is often still an issue. Typically they will describe poor concentration, with difficulty paying attention to something for more than a short time. If they try to push on through then they feel exhausted, as if their brain is shutting down. This cognitive fatigue is very disabling: somebody may get one or two paragraphs into reading an article or an email and feel themselves conking out. They will often be slow to process information. Once they start to venture outside they find that the cognitive overload of a busy street or a noisy pub will cause them to feel overwhelmed.

Such patients often struggle with executive function, which is an umbrella term for the cognitive skills that allow you to organise yourself. They will be irritable, an issue which tends to be flagged by their partner – 'He has rather a short fuse, doctor' – and sleep may be disrupted. Their mood will often be low and this will be made worse by experiencing failure when trying to get back to previous activities. There are often physical symptoms as well, such as dizziness and headaches. If you look up 'concussion' you will find many of these symptoms listed, but they are pretty much universal to head injury regardless of severity: neurologists have moved away from the term as it is not very useful.

A recent large survey of people in Europe six months after traumatic brain injury showed that 90 per cent of those with moderate or severe injury still had rehabilitation needs, and yet only 30 per cent had received any specialist input as an inpatient and 15 per cent as an outpatient. The majority had no input at all. This stores up big trouble for later on: those who carry this largely invisible disability out of the hospital door may find their lives falling apart as jobs and relationships fail. Alcohol often becomes a feature. A study of 8,000 male prisoners in Scotland in 2025 found that over 80 per cent had suffered a severe head injury at some point in the past. A similar proportion of women prisoners had been hospitalised with a head injury, in most cases more than once and often at the hands of an abusive male partner. This is not just a Scottish issue – similar figures have come out of Canada and New Zealand.

Those who find their way to prison must presumably be the tip of an iceberg of social disruption experienced by this group, and by those they encounter. A large recent study of the homeless population in Canada, incorporating almost ten thousand people, found a lifetime head injury prevalence of over 50 per cent. More than half of these injuries would have been categorised as 'mild' by current criteria, and in a recent study around 90 per cent of injuries pre-dated the period of homelessness. If you look further down the line, things get even worse. One study found that by thirteen years after brain injury over 40 per cent of their sample group were dead.

These are jaw-dropping figures. The missed opportunity to engage these walking wounded patients in rehabilitation early on and to offer them support sets off a ticking time bomb of social and medical problems to come. At the moment the mechanisms are simply not in place to pick these patients up after they are discharged, and if they are seen then the availability of rehabilitation outside hospitals is scarce. It is simply not considered to be a priority.

The link between brain injury and risky behaviour is well

established, but the chicken can at times be hard to separate from the egg. A man I looked after in his thirties was transferred back to the UK having suffered a severe head injury while on a boys' trip to Dublin – his post-traumatic amnesia lasted several weeks and in fact he had no memory at all of being abroad. He had jumped out of a moving bus for a laugh and landed on his head. I must have looked a little puzzled when he told me this so he clarified that one of his favourite hobbies was 'jumping off stuff': he seemed generally to relish a degree of peril in his life. He told me that he used to get in a lot of fights when he was at school, and when I dug into the details several of these had resulted in what would have been called at the time a severe concussion. So who is to say whether the thrill-seeking caused the brain injuries or vice versa?

For Vikas there did not seem to be any such prior tendency but of course the alcohol history indicated a degree of self-destructive behaviour which did ultimately contribute to the injury. Our neuropsychologists dug into how things had come to this point, speaking at length with both Vikas and his family. He had struggled with feelings of low mood since his teens but tended to cope by using alcohol. He kept his symptoms to himself and never sought help until drink became an obvious problem. He then dried out, but with the underlying depression undiagnosed the cycle kept repeating.

Vikas's cognitive difficulties fit closely the typical profile seen after head injury. Many functions were working well: his short-term memory had improved to a degree, his language was good, visuospatial skills were intact and his social skills were fine. The tasks he struggled with were those needing concentration over a period of time, planning and problem solving – those executive functions again. His working memory was also reduced and as a result he would only be able to encode a proportion of the information he was handling into longer-term memories.

We began to look at expanding Vikas's horizons beyond the hospital walls and the therapy team set a goal of planning a trip out into the real world. Libby joined him one morning along with neuropsychologist Monica, in one of the larger clinical rooms. They sat at a round table with a blank sheet of paper and a computer while the late summer sunshine poured in through the windows high above. Vikas was in his wheelchair but the hospital pyjamas were long gone and today he wore an indie band T-shirt with rather smart cargo trousers (harder to get on than tracksuit bottoms, but Vikas had standards). The wispy beard had gone, which made him seem younger but also brought out his hollowed cheeks.

Libby explained the parameters for the trip: it should be doable within three hours of an afternoon, it had to include public transport and it should be something he would find fun. What did he think? Vikas looked blank.

'So what should we do?'

'That's up to you, Vikas,' said Libby. 'It can be anything you want – as long as we can do it within an afternoon.'

He said nothing for a while, shuffled in his wheelchair and looked a little worried. The clinical room sits next to our main gym, and sounds of Heart 80s radio, whoops of encouragement and bouncing gym balls invaded the quiet. Then he smiled.

'Can we take Louise to the playground in our local park?'

Louise was Vikas's three-year-old niece and early on he had flagged taking her to the playground as a priority goal for once he left hospital. His brother had been bringing Louise in to visit at weekends but this was not the same: their local park would feel like real life again. The problem was that they all lived quite a way across London.

'That's a really nice idea, Vikas,' said Libby. 'Do you think we could get there and back in the time we have?'

'Probably, I reckon.'

'Well, if we are planning the trip then we need to work it out. How might we do that?'

Vikas was unsure initially but with a bit of prompting he suggested using a computer to look up the journey time, though he had trouble actually doing it. It was not easy for him to use the keyboard (he was once again surprised that his left arm would not bend) and when it came to the departure point he could not remember the hospital's name. Once the search result came up on the screen he seemed overwhelmed by all the information and needed help from Monica to select the right link. It turned out that it was going to take an hour and a half each way by bus (the tube is largely wheelchair-unfriendly). Vikas realised that this was not going to be feasible within the time they had but deferred again to Libby and Monica for help finding an alternative. They asked if he liked crazy golf. He thought this was a great suggestion and together they looked into travel times to the nearest course and other logistics: would it be wheelchair accessible? What were its opening times?

As a trio they worked their way through these questions but Vikas needed constant scaffolding for each step and as the session progressed he became increasingly anxious.

'You're putting me on the spot. I can't do it.'

They reassured him that he definitely could do it but it was taking longer than he would previously have expected. With time he would manage it. It had taken just under an hour to reach this point and Vikas's ability to concentrate was flagging so they stopped and set him some homework. He should speak to his physio about the physical considerations of playing crazy golf, and he should phone the course to confirm their hours and accessibility. He also needed to find a slot in his therapy timetable to complete these tasks.

By the end of the session Vikas had cheered up and was excited enough to call his partner and tell her about the crazy golf plan. It took a lot out of him, though, and before lunch he needed a lie-down to recover his energy for speech therapy in the afternoon.

*

Charles Symonds and William 'Ritchie' Russell were two British neurologists (both from the Queen Square stable) who in the inter-war years were among the first to study recovery from head injuries. They described the classic syndrome of post-traumatic amnesia based initially on observations of the many injured soldiers who had returned from the First World War. Symonds wrote in 1928 that instead of recovering rapidly, a more severely injured patient enters an altered state for days or weeks: '. . . he remains stuporose, restless and irritable. During the daytime, if left to himself, he is usually drowsy, lies curled up on his side, and resents interference. At night he is frequently noisy, hallucinated and violent.' Russell eventually collected a cohort of over three thousand soldiers with head injuries running right up to the Korean War, and with neurosurgeon Hugh Cairns and others did much to establish head injury rehabilitation as a field of study.

Symonds and Russell indicated that the duration of this amnestic period predicts the likelihood of a favourable outcome. This continues to be the cornerstone of prognostication even now: a study in 2009 found that for patients with post-traumatic amnesia lasting between one day and two weeks there was a 70 per cent chance of returning to productive employment by one year. This drops to less than 20 per cent for durations of four weeks or more, each additional week further reducing this probability. But while this model works well at a group level, it is less accurate for individual patients. Even Symonds and Russell cautioned against making predictions on this basis, noting that the point at which amnesia ends is hard to define as memory often fluctuates for a period as patients emerge from the fog.

In the hours and days after the initial injury the surviving brain tissue suffers a secondary insult similar to that seen after oxygen deprivation, with swelling, raised pressure and a build-up of toxic metabolites all making things worse. Overactivity of the brain's neurons can also feed into this vicious cycle, a process known as 'excitotoxicity'. ICU doctors will often put the patient into an induced coma for this stage and will rigorously control metabolic conditions to minimise this injury, focusing on blood glucose, oxygen and carbon dioxide levels, blood pressure and temperature. In theory, medications could be used to reduce the secondary injury after trauma, mopping up toxic metabolites, suppressing inflammation or calming overactive neurons. This approach has indeed been beneficial in animal models of traumatic brain injury, but frustratingly, other than a few small studies, none of these treatments have so far shown any significant benefit for human patients.

While most of the post-traumatic inflammation settles down within weeks there is one cell type which remains active, whose significance is unclear at the moment. Our brains contain small scavenger cells called microglia whose job is to swallow up and clear away any cellular debris which is clogging up the works. These usually lie dormant, but after a head injury the microglia switch on, remaining activated in animals and humans for months or even years. Opinions differ as to whether they are supporting recovery or instead perpetuating a harmful inflammatory state: for now nobody knows quite what these microglia are up to.

In the surrounding intact brain tissue there is plenty of evidence in the early stages after traumatic injury of cellular changes similar to those I have described after stroke, such as axonal sprouting and dendritic branching. These are the hallmarks of neuroplasticity, which is likely to be supporting recovery also following traumatic injury. This is an important insight for treating patients like Vikas: it means that all of the principles we use to drive neuroplasticity and promote recovery after stroke can be applied equally to traumatic brain injury.

Genetic factors may also be important in recovery. A large 'genome-wide association study' of 5,000 head injury patients in 2021 found that around a quarter of the variance in outcomes can be explained on the basis of genetic make-up, and a few specific genes may predict a patient going on to develop dementia. As with almost any condition you care to study, the biology of head injury is likely to reflect an interaction between genes and the environment.

*

Libby took Vikas to the therapy kitchen for his first attempt at cooking. At a table in the corner sat Jeremy, who was slowly making himself a jam sandwich, and as they came in he looked up and smiled. He was a different man recently. After weeks of relentless, strained positivity his wife Lauren had finally collapsed in tears with one of the therapy team, sharing her fears of years to come spent as a carer and her distress at the loss of the perfect gentleman she had married. Jeremy was not lost, of course, but was certainly different, and Lauren was beginning to understand the change. This shift had been like a weight off his shoulders and Jeremy was now relaxing into his rehab and starting to make progress.

Vikas, meanwhile, was excited at the prospect of producing a meal and had suggested a recipe from his French cookery book, a stew which he wanted to make for the other men in his bay. Libby felt it would be better to start with something a little simpler and he had reluctantly agreed, so they got hold of some burger patties and buns. She took his hand and helped him up from his wheelchair onto the high perching stool.

'Right, Vikas, what do we need to make this burger?'

He listed the ingredients – they were going all out on onions and relishes – but could not then say where to find them. She prompted him to look in the fridge for some things and in the cupboard for others. Having gathered these he was able to use both hands to open the packet of buns – leaning his half-flexed left arm on the Formica surface to hold the packet and using his right hand to pull at it – but when it came to chopping onions he needed Libby's help to stabilise them and to grip the knife tightly enough. The hob would not turn on. Vikas turned the dial, sat and waited but nothing happened so Libby asked whether the main switch was on at the wall. Having fixed this he put a glug of oil into the pan and got the patties going.

As the burgers began to sizzle Vikas hummed happily to himself. But almost immediately he tried, rather unsuccessfully, to turn them over using a wooden spoon so Libby asked him what the best implement would be. Once armed with a fish-slice he started impatiently to flip the burgers while they were still pink and falling apart, and she had to remind him a few times to wait. One of the other patients was making toast in the corner and soon Vikas was chatting away to him. A happy mood took hold of him as he began to assemble the other elements of his lunch, but while he was focused on this the onions began to catch and Libby had to intervene. By now Vikas had forgotten about the burger patties entirely and again Libby had to remind him to rescue them when a strand of smoke drifted up towards the ceiling. Having taken the pan off the hob he then held it too far down the handle and burnt his index finger. Libby ran his hand under a cold tap but Vikas dropped the pan into the sink with a crash. By now he was struggling to keep it together. His breath was coming fast and a film of sweat was forming on his brow. Libby turned everything off and they both sat down to get their breath back. Once the smoke had cleared and they had established that Vikas's finger was only slightly scalded Libby helped him to salvage some passable burgers to have for lunch.

The session had not been the confidence builder Libby had hoped for but it had highlighted the difficulties Vikas was having with maintaining attention and multi-tasking. When I passed by his bay that afternoon I found him sitting by the bed staring bleakly into the middle distance. I had not yet heard about burgergate and asked him how the kitchen session had gone. He said nothing and indicated with his left hand the slightly charred remnant on his plate. I saw that he was unable to speak and as I perched on his bed his eyes pricked with tears.

'Bloody useless, aren't I. Can't even cook a bloody burger.'

He picked up the Elizabeth David book and handed it to me.

'You might as well put this in the bin.'

By now he was crying properly. I told him that what he was trying to do was extremely hard and takes time – people often take months just to manage the basics of looking after themselves. Cooking is the ultimate cognitive test and perhaps we had tried this a little soon: two steps forward and one step back is pretty standard. In the grand scheme of things, he was doing well. He nodded but still he could not speak for a while and I took him to the day room for a cup of hot chocolate.

Vikas bounced back well, buoyed by some progress in physiotherapy and a more successful kitchen session the following week. We began to make arrangements for him to spend a day at home with his mother and partner at the weekend, and to think about what sort of support he would need once he left hospital. It was his mother's birthday in two weeks' time and the aim was for him to spend the night at home after a celebratory family dinner. In order to make this happen the therapists needed to make sure that his family knew how to manage the wheelchair, check that Vikas could get in and out of the bathroom and assess the risks involved in an overnight stay at this point. We decided to go ahead.

*

Since patients with traumatic brain injury have been followed up for longer and in larger numbers it has become apparent that there is also a longer-term issue: some will go on later to develop dementia. As more of us live longer than our three score years and ten, and since conditions such as Alzheimer's disease relate very clearly to age, the incidence of dementia is of course increasing in any case. But it is now clear that a brain injury presents a significant further risk of this happening: a study based on a Swedish national database suggests that even a mild injury increases your dementia risk by a factor of 1.6, while others have found an increase of up to three times. This is a difficult area of study and it can be hard to disentangle the long-term cognitive effects of a previous injury (superimposed on the effects of ageing) from a subsequent dementia. But there is an increased risk also of Parkinson's disease and it does now seem that brain trauma can in some people trigger a neuro-degenerative process to take place.

For repetitive head trauma this has been known for years and the phenomenon of the punch-drunk boxer was first described in the 1920s. Later termed 'dementia pugilistica', this incorporated a progressive cognitive decline but also physical symptoms such as slow movement and poor balance. This field of enquiry has more recently been turbo-charged by the realisation that people who engage in even fairly standard contact sports such as rugby or football are also at risk of early onset dementia. Given that there are somewhere around three million sports-related concussions each year in the US alone, you can imagine the concern.

If you measure the brain volumes of patients with previous head injury – a literal volume, calculated from MRI scans and measured in millilitres – you find that these shrink on average by 1.5 per cent each year. To put this in context, volume reduces by 0.5 per cent annually beyond our mid-thirties with normal ageing (whatever that is) and by 2 to 3 per cent in Alzheimer's disease. The rate of volume loss correlates with markers of head injury severity such as post-traumatic amnesia duration as well as with measures of cognitive function. This brain atrophy makes more sense since the discovery in autopsies of a characteristic abnormality in this patient group, now known as the Chronic Traumatic Encephalopathy (CTE) body. This resembles in some respects one of the classic pathological findings in Alzheimer's disease – the neurofibrillary tangle – in that it is made of the same kind of protein known as hyperphosphorylated Tau. At present the only way to detect CTE bodies is under the microscope – there is no scan – so in humans this is usually only possible at autopsy. Once people started looking, however, it became apparent that they are found in all sorts of situations where people have been exposed to repeated low-level head trauma: contact sports, physical abuse and retired military who have experienced blast injuries.

The Tau protein is an increasingly important character in the developing story of neurodegenerative diseases and is the hallmark of several conditions all now grouped together under the umbrella term Tauopathies. Tau is a relatively short protein, small enough to be soluble, which seems to play a role in holding together the microtubules within neurons. Microtubules are long hollow rod-like structures that run along our neurons' axons, where they make up part of the physical structure but also provide the means by which proteins made in one part of the cell can be transported to another. The normal forms of Tau protein (we have six kinds) are soluble, so if they become detached from their microtubules then they are simply recycled. If, however, its form has been altered slightly then it may detach from the microtubules and attach to other Tau proteins. If this happens then the Tau fragments will aggregate into larger and larger molecules, forming insoluble filaments and then larger tangles. These tangles get in the way of the mechanisms that keep the neuron healthy and ultimately lead to cell death. How trauma to the brain leads to alteration of Tau proteins – and ultimately to the formation of tangles, cell death and brain atrophy – is not yet understood.

The question of how post-injury dementia develops is more than a theoretical curiosity. We are entering a new phase of treatments for conditions such as Alzheimer's disease in which the abnormal amyloid – the protein which accumulates in the brain as part of that condition's pathology – can be gradually removed from the brain in living patients. These new treatments consist of synthetic antibodies which attach to the amyloid and target it for removal by our immune system, and while there is a way to go, it certainly looks like a promising approach. If we could identify head-injured patients who are at particular risk of neurodegeneration then such a strategy could present an opportunity to prevent this from happening. Given the numbers of patients with head injury, this seems something worth striving for.

*

Vikas's mother came to see me. I sat with her and Libby one afternoon after ward round in one of the clinical rooms. She was upset, and Libby closed off the viewing panel in the door as we pulled three chairs into a makeshift circle. A short Welsh woman with tightly cropped grey curls and a discreet pearl necklace, she clasped a handbag on her lap as she sat with eyes closed and gathered herself. With a dark cardigan over a floral dress she had the tidy look of someone who had been keeping things together at home for some time, and her eyes looked tired.

'This is harder than I thought it would be, doctor.' She dabbed her eyes with a tissue. 'For years I've managed Vikas, and I thought he was getting better. But now this.'

I asked how the weekend at home had gone.

'Don't get me wrong, it was lovely to have him back. Of course. But it was difficult. It's his brother Amit – he just doesn't get it.'

Her birthday dinner had been a success at first and Vikas was able to join in and chat with his partner and family. For a while they felt like they had Vikas back. But then after supper his brother had tried to persuade Vikas to come with him to their local pub. He had seen Vikas joining in at dinner, walking independently about the house and even helping to clear the table – he could not see why the pub would be any different. Vikas's mother had told Amit that he was not ready, it would be too much, and this had led to an argument.

'He sees Vikas chatting away and thinks he is just the same as he was. But he's not. Not by a long shot. And it's coming up to nine months now.'

She dissolved again. Libby and I tried our best to comfort her but she could see Vikas's future panning out and it looked very different to that she had wanted for him. His dreams of high-level French cooking seemed a long way off now.

We pointed out to her how far he had come over the last few months. The key was going to be continuing a rehabilitation approach after going home, so that once he was settled back into a routine and able to look after himself he could begin to think about getting back out into the world again and maybe even consider some form of work. This could all come with time if he had the right structures around him, and we were looking into whether we could arrange funding for a brain injury-trained carer to spend a few hours with him each day once he was discharged. The idea that Vikas's progress would continue after leaving hospital seemed to cheer her. She had been propping him up in various ways since long before this injury – in some ways this was a continuation of years of her caring role. She brought herself up straight in the chair and smiled.

'It'll be good to have help from people who know about this. Thank you.'

One aspect of Vikas's injury was a definite positive. He had really taken his mental health in hand and worked hard for months with our team to address the underlying mood issues which had festered for years. Vikas himself had described the whole process, grim as it was, as an opportunity for a reset and was keen for further psychology input after leaving hospital. He was not going to let himself slip into the deep end again. Vikas 2.0.

CHAPTER EIGHT

THE FAIRGROUND MIRROR

Sitting with my morning coffee, I find myself anchored within a world of which I am a part. A world to which I am central, in fact, at least as far as I am concerned. Feeling my fingers wrapped around the cup's handle and my bottom on the chair, I am aware of a boundary between myself and my surroundings, a line between where I end and the world begins. Visually, however, this frontier is less obvious. I cannot see my own eyeballs as I peer out of them and I have the impression of being in continuity with the room around me.

There is a familiarity to this world and how it behaves. I know which way is up and which is down. The second hand on my kitchen clock ticks in an even and regular fashion. From down the corridor I hear a click followed by rustling then another click. From prior experience my internal model of the world knows that this sound is my son who has come back for his forgotten sports kit: I can picture him now legging it down the street. I have the impression of inhabiting a predictable Cartesian world of which I am seamlessly a part.

But this cannot really be the case. For a start, the light that enters my eyes projects an upside-down and inverted image onto my retina like a pinhole camera but I do not perceive a topsy-turvy world. My coffee cup is not hurtling towards the ceiling. Some sort of transformation must have taken place between the world as it arrives in my brain and my perception of it.

The fact that I make such transformations without being aware of them suggests that to some extent I am actively constructing my perception of the world. Immanuel Kant suggested in his *Critique of Pure Reason* that we possess innate mechanisms by which we interpret our surroundings, that our perceptions must arise from an 'imaginative synthesis' of the information we receive. He argued that we are born with these faculties, rather than their being shaped by the outside world. He called this 'a blind though indispensable function of the soul . . . of which we are only seldom even conscious'. Over two hundred years later, this description of sensory perception has largely survived the discoveries of modern neuroscience.

As Gary discovered first hand, the constructed nature of the realities we each inhabit becomes frighteningly apparent when the mechanisms supporting them go wrong. He was outwardly healthy and only months before had taken a delayed retirement from decades of work as a trusted local estate agent. But Gary's coronary arteries had been quietly narrowing and one day while walking down the street a heart attack triggered a cardiac arrest out of the blue. Passers-by rallied round and started CPR, and after around fifteen minutes paramedics managed to get his heart restarted. At the hospital Gary gradually surfaced, but as he did it became apparent that he had suffered a stroke in the process: his left side was not moving at all and his eyes were fixed over to the right. Sure enough, a CT later confirmed a sizeable area of affected brain incorporating all of the right middle cerebral artery's territory.

Age spared Gary the need for surgery – by seventy-odd our brains have usually shrunk enough to allow for a little post-stroke swelling – and I first met him on our ward some weeks later.

Uroosa had briefed me on her assessment, so a day after his arrival we went and found him in the gym. His physiotherapist, Laura, had used a mobile hoist to get Gary from his tilting chair onto a plinth and had co-opted one of her colleagues, Rory, to help stabilise him in a seated position.

The gym was in full swing that morning. All of the plinths were in use, the thera-bikes were pumping away and in the corner a group of patients and therapists from the Upper Limb programme were working on assorted fiddly tasks. Our gym and our day room sit in the original part of the hospital building and were built according to the Victorian model with high ceilings, long windows and wide-open floors. If I could have stepped back into that era I would have seen Sir Victor Horsley himself – the world's first ever neurosurgical consultant, iconoclastic scientist and all-round good egg – performing pioneering brain surgery in this very room. Today sunlight poured in from the square, the radio supplied the soundtrack – Heart 80s, as usual – shoes squeaked on the floor and sweat was in the air. Far from a reverent silence, it resembled a scene from *Fame*.

We found Gary perched on the plinth's edge propped between Laura and Rory. His right leg was pushing hard into the floor and his whole right side was conspiring to arch his body leftwards: Laura and Rory were having to work quite hard to keep him upright. Uroosa and I greeted him, and with this distraction the pushing eased off for a while. Gary looked up and seemed momentarily surprised to find two doctors standing before him, then he smiled and grabbed onto my arm with his right hand. He was an expansive character with a good head of salt-and-pepper hair and a white beard over a strong jaw. He had the quizzical look of somebody who was on the verge of telling a joke, which it turned out he often was. I could imagine him holding court at the golf club bar.

The first thing that struck me on meeting Gary was the gross asymmetry between the two halves of his body. His left arm sat inert on his lap, but what that side lacked in movement his right side more than made up for with an almost comical excess of activity. His right foot pawed the ground as if he was constantly about to stand up. The right side of his trunk pushed him into occasional dives to the left, which Laura was at pains to resist. But it was his right arm which was most remarkable: as we talked it seemed to have an agenda entirely of its own, and a busy one at that. His hand grabbed at my arm, clawed its way up to my shoulder, let go of that and found Uroosa's leg instead. We put his hand back onto his lap but it was quickly off again, this time fiddling with his tracksuit bottoms. Gary seemed entirely unaware of what his errant arm was doing – when we brought his attention to it he laughed as if it were a magician's novelty trick.

Gary very strikingly ignored everything on his left side. When I asked him where Laura was (she was propping his trunk up from the left) he could not find her. I could direct his attention briefly to a sensation on his left – a tickle of his left leg, for example – but if I touched both sides then he would only notice the right. Gary seemed unaware even of his own body on that side. When we asked him to show us his left arm he could not do it and looked around as if perplexed. We lifted his arm up, placed his left hand in front of his eyes and asked him what this was.

'I don't know. It's not mine. Is it your hand?'

Gary seemed, if anything, slightly amused at this ridiculous limb which did not seem to belong to anyone and he shrugged it off with a laugh – he showed a gross perceptual distortion affecting the world around him but including even his own body. Christian the bartender had suffered from this hemispatial neglect (or inattention – there are a number of overlapping names) to a lesser extent. Although Gary was manifesting it particularly severely it is in fact pretty common, affecting in some studies well over half of patients in the early stages after right-sided stroke.

In hemispatial neglect there is a reduced ability to pay attention to one side of space even if there is no actual loss of sensory input. Somebody might be able to feel or see on the affected side if this is tested specifically but will tend to ignore it. As a result they may bump into things on their left side or only put their arm through one sleeve of their shirt when getting dressed. This asymmetry is often noticed by others rather than by the patient, who by definition is largely unaware of the issue. When the occupational therapists started to get Gary into the bathroom, he shaved only the right side of his face and declared himself finished.

When neglect is severe then it is easy to detect, but we always look for it when there is damage to one of the cerebral hemispheres. We give the patient a piece of paper covered in stars, letters and other shapes, and ask them to draw a line through all of the small stars with a pencil. When they say they are done we count the number of small stars they have missed. Gary managed to catch eight stars on the extreme right but missed all of the other forty or so. I asked him if he was sure he had finished: he took another look and told me that he had. On a fresh sheet I then drew four horizontal lines of differing length and asked him to put a mark at the halfway point of each. All of his marks were well over to the right as he was failing to perceive the left half of each line. No matter what test we used, Gary scored in the severe range.

Neglect crept rather gradually into the neurology literature. In early descriptions it was often seen in the context of grosser disorders of one side of the brain and so was hard to distinguish as its own entity. In 1876 John Hughlings Jackson described a woman with a right parietal tumour, whose impairments he summarised as 'left hemiplegia and imperception', in which hemispatial neglect appears to have been present alongside wider visual and motor difficulties. But it was the splendidly named Walter Russell Brain who first proposed neglect as its own disorder when in 1941 he described three patients, all with differing pathologies involving the right hemisphere – one tumour, one haemorrhage and one brain abscess – but who shared the odd property of preferring the right side to the left. As the first tried to evacuate from his London home during wartime air-raid warnings he would get lost: he headed downstairs aiming for the sitting room but 'tended to turn to the right instead of to the left and in consequence would arrive in the dining room'. This patient described that he 'did not know where the left side of his body was'.

None of these people had 'pure' neglect in that all three also showed other impairments. One woman also reported that 'a little Chinaman came and sat on the end of her bed'. But Brain was clear in distinguishing an impairment of attention to one side of space from the other symptoms such as visual loss or weakness. If we lose vision to one side then we would usually compensate by turning our head to take in the whole scene, but these patients were not managing to do this.

Since these original descriptions the phenomenon has been explored in detail and found to be quite heterogeneous in that different aspects of perception or even movement may be affected. Gary showed neglect with respect to his own body when shaving or dressing and particularly in his failure to identify his own arm, so-called asomatognosia. His left leg, unlike his left arm, had reasonable power, but when the physios started to stand him up he showed motor neglect: they needed repeatedly to remind him to bring that leg into play.

Neglect further afield may be less obvious. You might ask a patient to list ten objects in the room around them and find that they fail to include anything to one side. They may fail to notice sounds from one side of the ward. Once patients start to move about this usually becomes more apparent: I have lost track of the number of times the left side of a door frame has been damaged by a power chair.

Intriguingly this spatial bias can extend also to our internal worlds. If you use an eye movement tracker to follow visual searches then it is unsurprising that patients with hemispatial neglect will tend to favour one side over the other. But a study which did this during the rapid-eye-movement phase of sleep in a patient with neglect found that the same was also true then – he was dreaming more to the right than to the left.

One description of this 'representational neglect' illustrates this particularly elegantly. Milanese neuropsychologists Edoardo Bisiach and Claudio Luzzatti interviewed in 1978 two elderly patients with right parietal lobe strokes and signs of neglect. Both were lifelong residents of Milan and they were asked to describe from memory what they would see if they stood at the west end of the Piazza del Duomo looking eastward towards the enormous cathedral which dominates that end of the square. Both gave a detailed account of the view but missed out several prominent features to the left. For the reverse view – imagining standing on the cathedral steps facing west – they did exactly the same, the neglected region having shifted with their perspective as they mentally turned around. When prompted with the missed landmarks, 'the few left-sided items were mentioned in a kind of absent-minded, almost annoyed tone'.

The second patient was a lawyer and also gave a mental account of his place of work. The same phenomenon resulted, including the omission of his beloved piano at which he reportedly sat playing for two hours each day on completing his work: 'I am sitting in a Savonarola chair, behind a carved Renaissance table; in front of me there is an unknown master's painting representing Jesus Christ's flagellation; I have many books, some armchairs, a chandelier . . .' This gentleman's description of his workplace makes me wonder whether I may perhaps exist in the wrong era, profession and country.

Gary's errant right arm was something of a puzzle, grabbing and pawing at things with an apparent life of its own. There is a well-recognised phenomenon called Alien Limb syndrome – usually in the context of stroke or some neurodegenerative conditions – where an arm can behave in this way. But this typically affects the arm on the opposite side to the damaged brain, whereas for Gary the abnormal movement was on the same side as his stroke and involved his strong arm. He also lacked the sense of estrangement from the moving arm that is part of that condition (though he certainly had this on the weak side), so this could not be Alien Limb syndrome. In fact we see a degree of overactivity of the strong side fairly commonly in patients with large strokes. I have puzzled over how this might come about, with colleagues who are expert in alien limbs. One suggestion is that the usual inhibition of the left hemisphere by the right is lost due to the large stroke, releasing excess activity from the intact side which takes a while to 're-balance'. Perhaps a better term for Gary's arm would be an anarchic limb.

So how does such a distortion of our spatial attention come about? And why is it usually the left side of space that is affected? Since Brain's original article the advent of functional brain imaging has thrown light on the networks supporting our attention mechanisms. The right parietal lobe is thought to house our spatial representations of the world – our map room. Patients with a stroke here often have difficulties with navigation, failing to find their way around even familiar spaces. So perhaps the right side of the brain is simply dominant for spatial attention, much as the left is for language, and this explains the asymmetry. But we now know that the attention network spans several parietal and frontal regions: neglect can result from damage to any of these, including sometimes on the left side.

A popular theory suggests that neglect results from an imbalance between the attention networks in the brain's two hemispheres, each of which is competing to push attention towards the opposite side of space – a so-called interhemispheric rivalry model. It seems that you can even upset this balance experimentally in healthy people by delivering a magnetic pulse over one parietal lobe. This interferes with normal function, causing people transiently to bias their spatial attention towards the stimulated side – if you stimulate both sides at the same time then no imbalance occurs. So, could neglect result from a loss of this normal balance? There is support for this idea both from animal models and in patients, including one case in which a patient's neglect following a right parietal stroke was subsequently 'cured' by a stroke on the other side. This model, though, would not on its own explain the tendency for neglect to occur after right-sided damage.

It has become apparent more recently that while neglect is by definition a disturbance of symmetry, there are elements which have nothing to do with spatial awareness. The same patients usually also show difficulties with sustaining attention, working memory and vigilance, functions which are unrelated to spatial location and which rely on connections between the parietal and frontal lobes. Hemispatial neglect probably includes both a side-dependent disruption of spatial awareness and a more general difficulty with focusing attention. The network which promotes vigilance and looks out for new stimuli sits mainly in the right hemisphere, so perhaps this explains neglect's right-sided bias.

*

As I walked through our day room I came across Gary eating his dinner. The evening meal is served horrifically early in hospitals for reasons that have more to do with logistics than with patients' desires. As far as I was concerned it was teatime. To his right at the small round table sat his wife, Coleen. She looked rather younger than Gary, a tidy woman with close-cropped brown hair whose ruddy cheeks suggested that she joined him often on the golf course. Their table was nearest to the TV which occupies one corner of the day room and around that time of day always seems to be showing classic Westerns of the sort that I associate with childhood Sunday afternoons. As it was in my line of vision I would have switched the TV off but one of the other patients was sitting by it, so I tried not to watch over Gary's head. A ragged posse was peering over the brow of a hill at a line of carriages passing through a dusty plain.

Gary greeted me warmly and I asked how his dinner was. He grinned.

'Nice, thanks. Spag bol and peas. Not exactly Gordon Ramsay but this is the NHS so what do you expect?'

Coleen pointed at his plate, rolled her eyes indulgently and laughed.

'He thinks he's finished!'

I looked down and saw that the right half of his plate had been scraped clean but the left still held a pile of peas and a good portion of spaghetti. It was as if somebody had drawn a line down the middle of it. I turned the plate around for him, bringing the other half of his dinner into his field of attention. He grabbed my hand, threw his head back and laughed.

'Ha! Well, what do you know? I thought they were being a bit tight with the rations. I'm a hopeless case, doc!'

I left them to it and, as I went on my way, Gary was attacking the remaining spaghetti with a fork, chuckling to himself and joking with Coleen against a backdrop of clattering wagon wheels and rifle fire.

Gary was making progress with basic mobility, but the therapists were telling me that neglect was still a major obstacle to his rehab. It just got in the way of everything they tried to do with him. Often the severity reduces over the first few months but in nearly half it will persist, at least to a degree. The mainstay of therapy involves drilling the patient to bring their attention back into the affected part of space, often training them to use horizontal scanning techniques such as the self-explanatory lighthouse strategy. But the patient needs to remember to do this and the very nature of neglect makes that difficult. It is a little like telling somebody with memory problems to be less forgetful.

A number of tricks have been tried as adjuncts to the standard approach, each an attempt to drag the patient's attention leftward: sounds produced to one side, a vibrating device applied to the left of the neck, prism glasses which make everything seem further to the right than it really is (forcing you to reset your attention leftwards). In smooth pursuit therapy, patients watch a large screen filled with objects drifting leftwards, inducing involuntary eye movements which drag your attention to that side. It is currently hard to deliver such therapies in a quantity likely to be effective, but this may change with cheaper immersive virtual reality.

If neglect results from an imbalance between the attention networks of the two hemispheres then it should be a prime candidate for brain stimulation. The idea is to use electrical or magnetic stimulation to suppress activity in the attention network of the non-stroke hemisphere and by doing this to push attention back towards the neglected side. Several researchers have tried this approach and it does seem that doing this can improve neglect symptoms in many patients, at least for a period of time after the treatment, and that in some the benefits can persist. At the moment this remains in the realm of experimental treatments, and in the weeks after a stroke there may be medical reasons why patients are not well enough to undergo this sort of procedure. The other issue is that stroke is such a heterogeneous disorder – in research studies any treatment effect will often get lost in the variability of patients and their strokes. One size does not fit all, and a more tailored approach may be necessary. As a result, articles reporting such studies often end with phrases such as 'More research is needed to determine . . .'

*

Gary was living inside a reality distortion field that was heavily skewed, his world pulled to one side as a star's gravity bends the fabric of space-time around it. For others, such disturbances of perception may instead affect the images of the world around them conjured up by their brains. We take a smooth visual scene for granted, but once the fabric of this visual reality is torn then we are back through the looking glass.

This was certainly true for Anton, the radiographer who came to us with patchy brain damage following a cardiac arrest. There were large gaps in his visual fields, holes that his brain filled with hallucinatory apparitions such as the mannequins that peered at him benignly but persistently when light conditions were low. But even where he did have vision, it was oddly distorted – there were parts of his visual fields where he could only see things if they moved, and even when he could recognise objects he had great difficulty separating a scene out into its component parts.

One of the first indications that visual processing is modular, with distinct areas of cerebral cortex analysing specific aspects of the visual world, came from a now classic description given by George Riddoch. A young Scottish doctor, he had plans to become a neurologist but was still in training when the First World War broke out. He was promptly appointed a temporary captain in the army and assigned to the Empire Hospital for Officers in London (now long gone, like its namesake), where he received casualties from far-flung battlefields. It was here in 1917 that he published a description of nine injured men with injuries to the back of the brain, each with an odd form of visual loss.

One such man 'was wounded on April 6, 1916 by a bullet in the right occipital region, while advancing into action with his men. He did not fall and though dazed carried on.' This stoic lieutenant did eventually pass out and woke up eleven days later in a hospital in Rawalpindi, by which time the bullet had been removed from his brain. Riddoch examined him about two months later, once he had been shipped back to Blighty, and made the following observation: 'I found that he quickly perceived finger movements in the whole of the left half field, though when the fingers were kept stationary he saw nothing; and, moreover, that the field for movement compared with my own was normal.'

Several of Riddoch's other patients showed a similar phenomenon and he concluded that 'Movement may be recognized as a special visual perception.' He was working in an era when doctors had the time to observe patients carefully over a number of months – now the patient would be discharged smartly and the doctor would be busy with admin. Accordingly he noted that 'Appreciation for movement returns before the object as such is recognized, if recovery of vision is occurring.'

More bizarre visual dissociations had been described the previous year by S. Smith and Gordon Holmes – also temporarily in uniform – in their account of a twenty-seven-year-old who had been injured in the first year of the war. Their patient was an engineer and draughtsman who had been shot in the top of his head while in action, the bullet entering from the right side and lodging just above and behind his left ear. He was dazed and confused for several days and had no memory of getting back to base but once more alert appeared remarkably unscathed. He had no weakness, was fully conversant (with a minor stutter which soon disappeared) and at a superficial level seemed intellectually intact. Smith and Holmes in their account were most interested in the difficulty he had manipulating objects with his hands – motor apraxia – but they also described a striking visual disturbance. Their engineer was unable to look them in the face when they stood before him. Nor could he look at or locate an object placed in front of him: '. . . when asked to do so, he generally stared open-eyed in a wrong direction, and then moved his eyes about in an irregular manner, most commonly towards the ceiling, saying "Sometimes I can see quite well, but often I cannot see what I want to look at."'

Once he had successfully located something he had no apparent difficulty in recognising it and there were no visual fields gaps for movement. But he was unable to follow a slowly moving finger and if asked to look at his own hand could not do so. He was observed trying to find a box of matches in his locker: he turned his head and eyes towards it, stared vacantly at one spot, then slowly and deliberately moved his eyes about until after a while the matchbox came into his central vision. He could then reach out to take it, though he missed at first attempt.

He could not determine the relationship between two objects, for example judging which was closer, or which of two lines was the longer. Expressing frustration, he stated, 'I can only look at one at a time.' He found it very hard to navigate his way around the ward and if brought into a large room would nervously walk across it before coming up against a chair. This would take him by surprise and he would side-step around it 'very much as a crab does when it meets a stone'.

This description from over a hundred years ago is strikingly similar to what we observed when Anton first started to walk around the ward. Likewise, if you held a pen in front of him and asked him to reach for it, he would often entirely miss. Something similar had been described in detail seven years before Smith and

Holmes's report by the Hungarian neurologist Rudolf Bálint in Budapest. His patient suffered a spontaneous stroke affecting the back of the parietal lobes on both sides and this left him with a similarly odd visual disorder. Bálint separated out the three key elements of this peculiar presentation – inability to locate a visual target, difficulty making voluntary eye movements towards something, inability to separate out visual elements – and it carries his name still.

Raw information arrives for processing right at the back of the occipital lobes in the primary visual cortex. Here it is laid out according to a very precise map of the visual world – in high resolution and corresponding closely with the retinas – with each neuron having a small visual area to which it responds (which we call 'a small receptive field'). From here the visual information passes forward to the secondary visual cortex where it is analysed according to parameters such as colour, edge detection and spatial orientation. As the information works its way forward across the cortex more complex visual features are extracted and the analysis becomes more abstract. Here we find neurons that are tuned for specific shapes or for motion in a given direction, and with increasingly large receptive fields. This process is analogous in some ways (though in reverse) to that for movement: motor commands start as abstract complex movements at the front of the brain and become more specific as they move backwards through the frontal lobes.

It is now thought that, broadly speaking, two streams of visual information flow through the cortex. The ventral stream works its way sideways towards the temporal lobes and is described as the 'what' pathway, operating relatively slowly to analyse and identify objects then linking to nearby emotional and facial recognition centres. The dorsal stream flows forwards and upwards and is known as the 'where' or 'how' pathway, operating fast to analyse spatial and movement characteristics of objects then passing this on towards movement centres to guide any responses. Each passing year neuroscience adds a little more complexity to this model but the overall principle still holds, with a ventral stream focused on perception and a dorsal stream focused on action.

It is interesting to consider at what point the information in these visual streams reaches the level of awareness, where it becomes something we are conscious of having seen. The nature of consciousness is its own can of worms, but when observing patients like Anton you do feel very close to the interface between the cold physics that we inhabit and the more magical perceived reality which our brains construct for us: when these systems are damaged a small hole opens up between these adjacent worlds. Peering through this torn corner of the canvas at the workings beneath does not for me detract from the grandeur of this perceptual conjuring trick. Unlike the Wizard of Oz, revealed by Dorothy to be but a petty illusionist cowering behind a curtain, we keep in our perceptual machinery an Old Master capable of transforming patterns of photons into visual poetry of sublime richness. To me this seems like magic.

*

Angela was in her early sixties, a petite and chatty social work assistant by day who cared for her unwell husband in the evenings. She came to us almost four months after bleeding from an aneurysm at the bottom of her brain. There were several areas of damage – patches of darkness on her CT scan – but the most prominent involved both of her occipital lobes. This included her primary visual cortex on both sides and as a result she could see nothing at all. She could just about perceive a bright light shone into either eye but beyond that could not make out anything. Testing her visual fields was impossible as she could not detect the target anywhere. Examining her eyes themselves revealed nothing amiss (confirmed by the eye clinic) because, of course, the problem was further back in the brain itself. Angela was cortically blind.

There was, however, a surprising finding when I examined her in more detail. If I sat facing her with my hands raised on either side she would not see them. If I wiggled my fingers then she was unaware that I was doing so. If I wiggled on one side only and asked her which side I had moved she would tell me that she had no idea – she thought it odd that I would even ask, seeing as she was blind. But I asked her to guess anyway and found that mostly she would get it right – she was consistently 'guessing' the correct side. The same was not true if I asked her to locate a stationary hand. When I pointed this out she initially thought I was joking and then was very surprised. I asked her what she experienced when I moved my hand: she told me she was not aware of anything at all. The visual information about movement was somehow getting through but not at a conscious level.

This 'blindsight' has been recognised as an unusual but real phenomenon since it was described in the 1970s by American psychologist Larry Weiskrantz at the University of Oxford, working with Elizabeth Warrington at my hospital. More typically this is seen when vision has been lost on one side only. Weiskrantz and Warrington reported a patient whose right visual cortex had been removed in surgery. He had no functioning vision on the left but could accurately reach towards a target suddenly presented in the blind area with a hit rate that was well above chance. Again he had no awareness of 'seeing' anything.

The question of what blindsight means for conscious experience has stirred its share of controversy. My colleague Sara Ajina studied seventeen patients who had lost their primary visual cortex on one side, either from stroke or tumour surgery, and had a blind opposite visual field. Twelve of these patients showed definite blindsight in the affected field – they could detect a moving shape at an above-chance level without 'seeing' it – while five did not. On detailed MRI brain scanning she found that what distinguished the blindsight group was the presence of an intact connection between the lateral geniculate nucleus (a relay station for visual information heading up to the cortex) and the part of the dorsal stream which is specialised for movement. The idea is that in patients with blindsight, information about movement is getting up to the dorsal stream (the 'where' pathway) via an alternative route which bypasses the damaged primary visual cortex. As there is no such connection to the ventral stream (the 'what' pathway), this remains cut off and the patient is unable to identify any object in the blind field.

For me the interesting question is why the perception of movement remains subconscious in these patients – why this information is in some way actionable and yet does not reach the threshold of awareness. Some neuroscientists maintain that for an incoming stimulus of any kind to generate conscious awareness it must trigger simultaneous activity across several regions spanning the brain, lighting up a network that is wide enough to meet the threshold for awareness. Others suggest that to be conscious of seeing something the information must complete a feedback loop from the higher regions to the primary visual cortex. At this point it all begins to get a little fuzzy and debates about what constitutes conscious awareness begin to make my own brain short-circuit.

In other patients we may see the opposite mismatch between visual perception and awareness. Somebody who is rendered cortically blind will sometimes behave as if their vision is normal and will flatly deny having any difficulty seeing. When challenged they will find other reasons for making errors – there is something in the way, the light is not good enough. They may give elaborate descriptions of what they are looking at as their brains fill in the gaps. I have seen this with strokes or bleeds like Angela's (though she was aware of her symptoms) and even with occipital damage from multiple sclerosis. This phenomenon was described originally by the Austrian Gabriel Anton, for whom it is named, and probably represents a visual form of the anosognosia – the lack of awareness of one's own impairment – that Babinski reported in his patients with weak left sides.

Patience showed a different and more disturbing derangement. A Nigerian woman in her fifties, she worked as a teaching assistant in a primary school and she came to us having bled from an aneurysm near the bottom of the brain. The blood had spread much of the way around the outside causing swelling of the hemispheres with patchy strokes around the brainstem, occipital and temporal lobes. She had difficulty using her right arm, but her most prominent symptom was a constant stream of visual hallucinations to her left. Patience saw brightly coloured fish swimming about on that side, which sometimes drifted across from left to right. These long fish resembled eels and did not look like those she used to see in the markets of Lagos growing up. The fish would dart about then swim at her and try to nibble her face, so she swatted them away with her left hand. She sometimes managed to squash one but although she would then see blood on her hand she would not actually feel anything.

We considered the possibility that this was Charles Bonnet syndrome – named for the eighteenth-century Swiss naturalist whose partially blind grandfather reported detailed visual hallucinations – where the brain's visual machinery constructs apparitions to fill in gaps. But Patience did not have a field defect: as far as we could tell she could see fully to both sides and could read well in the centre. Her visions also seemed to be much more intrusive and disturbing than the usually benign apparitions of Charles Bonnet, which tend to sit passively by like Anton's mannequins and were described by Oliver Sacks (who experienced them) as like watching a film. Another possibility was that they were a form of seizure from the right occipital lobe, but when we recorded the electrical activity from her brain during the visions we found nothing amiss.

We concluded that Patience was experiencing 'peduncular hallucinosis'. She had damage to the cerebral peduncle on the right side of her brainstem, a region that included the connection between her brainstem's arousal network and her lateral geniculate nucleus – the visual relay station mentioned in relation to blindsight. The theory goes that this connection usually keeps that route into the visual pathway suppressed while we are awake, insulating our visual machinery from whatever is ticking over in our subconscious. In peduncular hallucinosis the loss of this inhibition allows background activity from the rest of the brain to spill over into the visual pathways as it might when we are dreaming, causing visual perceptions on the affected side.

Patience was understandably distressed when the fish were very active and she would cover her head with a blanket in a vain attempt to get away from them. At the start of her admission Patience's hallucinations often got in the way of her being able to take part in therapy sessions. We considered using antipsychotic medication to suppress them but they began to settle on their own after a few weeks. After two months or so they were gone. Once the fish had left her alone Patience's rehab took off and eventually she got back to living at home with her son with a decent degree of independence.

A study of the perceptual distortions resulting from the damaged brain is not actually necessary to appreciate the constructed nature of our visual world, what Sacks called 'the theatre of the mind'. The influential Gestalt school of psychology in the early twentieth century considered visual perception and took as their starting point Kant's suggestion that our imaginative processes form a bridge between the information we receive and our perception. They used introspective methods and visual illusions in healthy people to show that we constantly use inherent perceptual mechanisms to construct our reality. Instead of – or perhaps as well as – building visual scenes bottom-up from their constituent parts, we apply mechanisms that 'expect' to see objects of certain kinds and extract common forms from the information received. Examples often given include seeing a whole circle when there are only fragments, or the face-vase illusion in which we can only see one or the other and our perception pops between the two. The psychologists in this tradition devised a number of 'Gestalt principles' by which our visual systems extract meaning from the world and which can give rise to optical illusions.

One of their important insights was that not only do the components of a scene determine how we perceive the whole but the reverse is also true: like the rows of dots on a migraine-inducing carpet which turn into lines when we step further back, our perception of the individual elements depends on what our brain is making of the whole scene. For this to be true information must be moving both up and down the perceptual hierarchy at the same time.

In this constructed reality it seems that time is also elastic. When I look up at my wall clock I invariably have the impression that the second hand freezes for a second or more before continuing to move. This 'chronostasis' is a recognised illusion and just before I arrived at John Rothwell's lab he and his student Kielan Yarrow conducted an ingenious experiment that showed it occurs because we freeze our perception of time while we are making an eye movement. They asked subjects to look from a fixed point towards a counter which started ticking as soon as their eye movement began. They then had to make a judgement about how long the digit on the counter remained before changing: they reliably over-estimated this time by the same interval it took for their eyes to reach the target. So it seems that when we make a planned movement we extrapolate our perception of time back to the start of the action. Our visual perceptive mechanisms are actively suppressed during eye movements and blinks, so this is perhaps a way of filling in the perceptual gap and providing an illusion of continuity. It seems that time is not as linear as we would perceive it. Yarrow concluded that his data painted a picture of 'conscious experience as an on-going often post-hoc reconstruction emerging from multiple cognitive systems'. Or put another way, the theatre of our mind has many players.

*

For somebody so impaired, Gary was doing well. His left arm still only had flickers of movement but his overactive right side gradually settled down and he began to sit straighter and even stand up with support. He now knew that his left arm was his. He began to go out to local shops and cafes and to make food in the kitchen. The neglect proved hard to shift at first but did gradually improve, and he was no longer dressing or eating to one side to such an extent.

The upbeat approach that Gary brought to his rehabilitation had been a joy to work with and as he became gradually more independent I could feel the positive effect this was also having on the therapy team. They made him a cake as his discharge approached and we all made a fuss. With me his mood only slipped once, as I caught up with him and Coleen at his bedside. Her golf course tan had faded and she was beginning to look a little apprehensive about Gary's return home. He was telling me about a golfing trip to Spain that before the stroke he had been planning as an anniversary present for the two of them. As he warmed to his theme my mind drifted to how somebody with hemispatial neglect plays golf. Would it be like teeing off into a strong cross-wind?

'Anyway, it doesn't look like I'll manage that now,' he finished, but as he said it his voice broke and he crumpled. He closed his eyes and let the tears come for a minute. As he recovered, Gary grabbed hold of my wrist.

'Don't leave it too late, doc.' He fixed me with his eyes. 'She kept telling me to retire so we can enjoy ourselves but I thought I'll just carry on a bit longer. Then this happens. Do the things you want to *now*!'

The moment passed and Gary perked up again quickly, his white-bearded grin soon back in action. But he had a point. Doctors are worse than many when it comes to soldiering on and it got me back to thinking about time perception. What was the opposite of chronostasis?

When I caught up with Gary in the clinic a few months later he had all sorts of projects on the go: reorganising family photos, building a new extension and getting more involved with his children's families. He had reluctantly let go of the golf trip plan.

'But I've just discovered a brilliant new sport, doc. Have you heard of wheelchair padel?'

CHAPTER NINE

THE SILENT LANDSCAPE

As a child I had a recurring dream of a birthday party. I wandered about a brightly lit sitting room, coloured balloons careening off the other children as they milled about, and hoovered up unattended chocolate Rice Krispie cakes and jellies as I went. I looked up at the adults chatting happily to each other and asked one of the mothers some question but she frowned as if she could not understand me. I tried again, more slowly this time, but as I spoke I realised that what came out of my mouth was gibberish. The woman looked puzzled again and now she said something to me, but although I could hear the sounds she made they seemed to make no sense: it was as if I was hearing an unfamiliar foreign tongue. By now a few of the adults had gathered around me in a circle and were all talking to me, but though I looked helplessly up at them I could understand none of it. I started to panic – what was wrong with me? I looked down at my hands and felt my own mouth to make sure all was in place but as I looked up again I had a terrible fright. The adults had no faces, just flat discs of flesh where their features should have been – mouths, noses and even eyes all gone. Heart racing, I pushed my way through the ghoulish crowd. I tried to call out for help but as I did I knew that nobody could understand me.

To communicate with others is central to the human experience, hard-wired into what makes us who we are. Literally, as it turns out. I would wake up from this nightmare but for some it is their daily reality. Tarek disappeared in the middle of a working day. He was in his late forties and ran his own construction firm so he spent his days shuttling his van between client meetings and site visits. When he failed to arrive home one evening his wife Shaheeda assumed he was caught up with work, but then one of his foremen called her and said that they had not seen him since that morning and he had missed several meetings. She called everyone she could think of but nobody had heard from him.

Tarek's parents had moved to the UK from Pakistan but he was London through and through, a 'geyser' whose haunts were the greasy spoon cafes of the city's market streets. He knew everybody and they all knew him, a trusted local figure, and as his business and young family grew he became busier and busier. To drop off the grid was simply not Tarek's style and Shaheeda knew immediately that something was up.

The police were not interested as he had only been gone for a few hours so she left the children with her sister and drove around all the sites she knew he was working on. She had no luck but then remembered that she could track his phone's location and this led her to a site she had not known about. She pulled up in front of a small terraced house in a quiet street and found the door slightly ajar. There were no functioning lights in the house and she had to use her phone as a torch as she picked her way through the dusty hallway to the kitchen at the back. Tarek was slumped against the wall, semi-conscious and unable to speak. Shaheeda called 999.

I met Tarek just over a month later. A blood clot had blocked one of the branches of his middle cerebral artery on the left causing a reasonably large stroke on that side. Being young (at least by my criteria), Tarek had little room to accommodate the subsequent brain swelling, so he had undergone a hemicraniectomy and had a left-sided skull defect which by the time he arrived with us was beginning to sag. I found him at the bedside, where he was sitting in a tilting chair with Shaheeda perched on the bed next to him. It was mid-morning and the other patients in his bay were all elsewhere, so we had the curtains drawn back and the place to ourselves. Tarek had a half-finished bowl of porridge on the tray table in front of him alongside a cup of tea, artificially thickened to prevent choking. A feeble autumn light was struggling in from the square but it was a half-hearted effort and we still had the lights on.

Even now they were a glamorous couple. Tarek was handsome in a barber shop photo kind of way: impossibly thick black hair (currently missing a patch from the surgery), intense eyes and five o'clock shadow. He had an easy charisma, locking eyes with me, smiling and shaking my hand. As Shaheeda told me the story of their journey to this point I observed that Tarek had no movement on his right side and was leant slightly over to his right in the chair. He had some shoulder pain on the right that we would need to look at, but Tarek's most prominent impairment was his lack of speech, and I focused on this. I started with an open question to test the waters. How was he feeling today?

'I'm, I'm erm . . .' He smiled, closed his eyes for a couple of seconds then tried again. 'I'm er. I'm fah. Why can't . . . Fuckin' 'ell! I'm fah! Fuck.'

'You're fine?' I suggested.

'Thassit yeah! I'm fah.' He laughed. 'Not though, am I?'

Leaving it open to start with, I asked if he knew what sort of place we were in.

'We, we . . . We . . . You know. Shit!'

He kept groping for the word but just could not reach it and gradually his good humour gave way to frustration. I took a blank sheet of paper and wrote three words on it: Home, Hospital, Hotel. I pointed to them each in turn as I went through them.

'Are we at home, in hospital or in a hotel?' He looked relieved and pointed at the middle option.

'We're at a hop, hop . . . fuck! Hoptal.'

We went through a similar process to establish if he knew what had happened to him: heart attack, accident or stroke? He was unable to make the right sound but he recognised the word stroke and was able to pick it out correctly. If I wrote out a whole sentence then he struggled to understand it but single words were fairly reliable. I gave him a verbal instruction – 'Please touch your nose' – and he could do this. I made it more complicated – 'Before pointing to the ceiling please touch your knee' – and then his understanding broke down. So comprehension was not perfect, but getting words out was his main issue. Giving him a pen and paper made no difference: he could make marks on the page using his non-dominant left hand but he could not write any words that made sense. The problem was not movement but language. This was expressive aphasia.

Often automatic social phrases are preserved and when we first greeted each other Tarek had in fact said 'Hi' to me. Swearing is likewise often not a problem and words that carry greater emotional weight may be easier to access. I asked Tarek how many children he had, and he perked up.

'Thah, Thah . . .' He raised three fingers on his left hand.

'Three children! Can you tell me their names?'

'Bah, bah, beh . . . Oh God! Beh!'

Shaheeda chipped in.

'Becky?'

'Yeah!'

He tried the next one but got completely stuck and as he did his shoulders started to shake. Shaheeda put her arm around him while his head dropped and the tears began to run down his cheeks. I apologised for upsetting him and told him that I was trying to understand which bits of his speech were working well and which were difficult. Tarek's stroke had damaged the language network which sits on the left side of the brain, in his case disrupting his capacity to produce language more than his ability to comprehend it. I explained that this had interrupted the connection between the ideas in his head and the words that represent them. Our speech therapists were going to spend a lot of time with Tarek working on this: it was still early days and we hoped to see some improvement.

In 1825 the French physician Jean-Baptiste Bouillaud correlated speech symptoms with post-mortem brain findings to suggest that the frontal lobes were important for speech. But it was another Frenchman, Pierre Paul Broca, who in 1865 reported a patient who was unable to produce any fluent speech – he could only say 'Tan' over and again – and who at autopsy proved to have an abnormality in a specific gyrus of the left frontal lobe. Four years later Broca published a more definitive report based on a series of such patients, suggesting the 'third frontal convolution' as the seat of articulate language.

Inspired by this approach, the Prussian physician Carl Wernicke investigated patients with a fundamentally different language disorder. Nine years after Broca's report he described a series of patients in whom the difficulty was one of language comprehension rather than production. Like Tarek, Broca's patients could understand a spoken instruction, while Wernicke's could not. While Broca's largely failed to generate any fluent speech, Wernicke's spoke quite freely but the content lacked meaning. Broca had localised the damage in his patients to the back of the left frontal lobe and Wernicke localised his to the top of the left temporal lobe.

These observations gave rise to a model of language that has held sway in some form or other ever since. This has the two key cortical regions for language processing sitting either side of the left Sylvian fissure, the large diagonal fold in the brain that you would see if you looked from the left side: Broca's area in the inferior frontal gyrus for language production and Wernicke's area in the superior temporal gyrus for comprehension. If you dissect the brain you find that these two regions are anatomically linked by a J-shaped white matter tract which swooshes around the corner of the Sylvian fissure, known as the arcuate fasciculus.

This deceptively simple model for language processing – two cortical regions joined by a white matter tract – is attractive because it allows us to predict what kind of difficulties should result from damage to a given region. As with almost everything in neuroscience it turns out to be a little more complicated – to be fair, it would be a little disappointing if nothing had changed since 1874 – but broadly speaking the main patterns of language disorder, or aphasia, do conform to this model. In real life it is rare to find pure expressive or receptive aphasia: brain injuries (and people) tend to be messier than textbooks, so most have a mixture of difficulties.

The side of the brain housing language is defined as its dominant hemisphere. This is on the left for 95 per cent of right-handed people and even for the majority of left-handers, so a dominant right hemisphere is pretty unusual. As a result it is often the case for stroke that aphasia will be accompanied by right-sided weakness.

About two weeks after Tarek's arrival he was joined in his bay by Dritan, diagonally across from him by the window. Superficially these two had similar difficulties – right-sided weakness and language impairment – but in terms of their ability to function they occupied different worlds. While Tarek seemed at ease in his skin the same could not be said of Dritan. He was thirty-odd but seemed younger. Pale and slight, his almost translucent skin stretched over a light frame. His hair was cropped short and he leaned forward in his bed clutching the bed rail with his left hand and peering about nervously, like a frightened mouse looking to dash back behind the dresser. On the left side of his neck and across both forearms were livid scars, long red lines daubed in parallel as if in a horrific parody of decoration.

Dritan had moved to the UK from Albania three years previously. He had never really assimilated and lived almost entirely within the community of his countrymen, sharing a flat with five or six others and working as a courier. He was a dedicated member of his family, kind and gentle by their account, and would regularly send money home to his mother and siblings. About a year before we met him he started calling home less often and then fell out of contact altogether. His older sister Sihana had moved to the UK some years before and lived on the Essex coast with her own family. She came to London to look for him and found that he had fallen in with the wrong crowd. They argued and Sihana returned home, hearing nothing more until she was phoned some months later from a London hospital. Dritan had been the victim of a knife attack, left for dead in an alleyway with potentially fatal wounds to his neck and arms. His attackers had damaged his left carotid artery and while it was repaired he had suffered a stroke, a blood clot dislodging and embolising into his left middle cerebral artery. Since his injury he had shown no verbal output at all.

The nurses had already been having some difficulties with Dritan. Dennis told me that though he was mostly placid he would suddenly become worked up, pushing staff away or banging the bed rails aggressively. The issue was communication: they simply had no way of knowing what he wanted at any given moment and were having to anticipate his needs, with mixed results. I witnessed one such interaction while Dritan was sitting quietly by his bed after breakfast. The healthcare assistant Michael was planning to help him get dressed but as he approached with a T-shirt Dritan looked up and began to fidget in his chair, a sudden animation coming over him like leaves lifted by a restless wind. He ground his teeth together, shook the tray table in front of him until the cup fell to the floor and made a low roaring sound. He was red in the face. Michael put down the T-shirt and calmly asked him what the matter was. Did he need the toilet? Would he like more breakfast? Was he in pain? Dritan made no eye contact with Michael and responded by shaking and nodding his head, inconsistent gestures that only led to further confusion. He began to pull on the bed rail and gradually it became apparent that he wanted to go back to bed.

At my first encounter I had made little progress in assessing Dritan's communication, even using my best bedside tricks, so instead I joined his speech therapist Laurel in their first session. As we arrived, Michael was offering Dritan menu choices for dinner. He looked at the sheet of paper, pointed at one of the lines of text and then pushed it away. He seemed to have indicated shepherd's pie. Having introduced herself, Laurel asked Dritan if he was a fan of pies. He made no reply so she changed tack with some simple yes/no questions. Was he in hospital? Was he at home? Was his name Alban? Did he have a sister? Dritan looked at Laurel as she asked her questions but he made no attempt to answer and appeared not to understand her at all. She picked up his left hand and moved it into thumbs-up or thumbs-down positions, prompting him to answer this way, but he could not follow what she was doing. She encouraged him to give a nod or shake of his head, or to point at 'yes' or 'no' written on a laminated sheet. No response. Dritan was unable to respond to a single-stage instruction, such as sticking out his tongue. Laurel enlisted the help of an Albanian interpreter, though we had been told that his English was good, but this seemed to make no difference.

Laurel's lack of success made me feel slightly better about my own unsuccessful efforts but augured a tricky time ahead in therapy sessions. Unlike Tarek, Dritan suffered from an almost complete failure of language, global aphasia. The only form of communicative intent we had seen from him was when he either pushed something away, or rocked or ground his teeth to indicate discomfort or frustration. Dritan was stuck inside my childhood nightmare.

*

Global aphasia implies loss of all three key elements of the left-sided network. In Dritan's case there was likely also some difficulty in shaping movements with his mouth, so-called apraxia of speech. Laurel wrote in her notes: 'Profound communication disability. Global aphasia with likely orofacial apraxia.'

She kept plugging away in subsequent sessions, taking Dritan to our 'communication gym' and exploring in detail every possible avenue for making contact. He could hold a pen and when she coaxed him to copy a circle he could eventually do it, but when she moved on to the next task he got stuck drawing wobbly circles over and over. She tried a noughts-and-crosses game: he picked up the pieces and looked at them but could not play the game with her. As she arrived for their third session he seemed to indicate the photos of his nephews and nieces on the wall above him, which Sihana had brought in. Laurel asked if she could look at the pictures and Dritan nodded. In the session she showed him two pictures, a cup and a comb. She asked him to point to the cup and he was able to do this most times. So something seemed to be getting through, but he still could not follow a simple instruction.

Dritan's complete disconnection made it hard for him to participate in many of the activities which lie at the heart of rehabilitation. Though Tarek lacked fluent speech he was nonetheless able to respond to those around him. He was now finding a few more words and was also learning to use gesture and facial expression to get his point across pretty effectively. In fact as a result of his natural sociability a kind of cafe society had sprung up on our unit. Walking through the day room I would find Tarek at the heart of a group of patients, usually men, sitting around one of the tables chewing the fat and guffawing over a newspaper. Dritan would sometimes be peripherally present but he could not join in and usually sat at his own table. Wrapped in a cocoon of silence, he cut a haunted and solitary figure.

One afternoon Dritan's family drove up to visit and I found him in the day room with Sihana and her two young boys. They had got hold of our games collection and chatted away as they tried to play with him, apparently unfazed by his lack of verbal response. They patiently set up a draughts board in front of him, made the first few moves on his behalf and then whooped with excitement as he used his left hand to make his own move. As I watched Dritan with his two nephews I observed that he looked them clearly in the eye as they spoke to him, nodded at times to their encouragement and followed the process of the game as they demonstrated it. Sihana caught me watching.

'Pretty good, aren't they?'

'Yes,' I agreed. 'It's a shame about labour laws or we'd hire them.'

Sihana smiled.

'Dritan is most close to my daughter Milla,' she told me. 'She is fourteen now but he used to look after her when she was little. They are great friends. She won't come and see him though – I can't persuade her. She finds it too upsetting to see him like this. Me too. I try to talk to him but it is impossible. He is my baby brother and I love him, but it feels like there is no connection – it is like trying to have a conversation with my cat. I just can't . . .'

She paused and gathered herself.

'But you know his real love? Music.'

I raised an eyebrow. 'Really?'

'Yes. Almost professional at guitar back home. Also piano. If you want to get him out of bed this is his great love.'

I thanked her and went to catch up with Laurel for an update. Progress had been slow. She had managed to get Dritan to sort cards with pictures on them into appropriate categories – animals in one column, food in another – showing at least that visual recognition was working and that he had basic semantic knowledge of objects. Using this approach she had established that he was aware of being in hospital, but when she tried to probe further the task broke down and he became frustrated. Still, this felt like progress of a sort. Meanwhile the physios and occupational therapists were having a worse time of it: when working on a task such as brushing his teeth, Dritan would quickly become overwhelmed and end up pushing them away with his arm. I told Laurel what I had discovered about Dritan's love of music. Perhaps we could somehow unlock his engagement this way? Laurel smiled. This was old hat: she had already referred him to our music therapist.

The fact that we see such distinct patterns of communication impairment across patients with differing brain injuries supports the idea that we process language in a modular manner. The great American linguist Noam Chomsky rejected the incumbent view in the 1950s and 1960s of human language as a learned behaviour that we simply absorb into a naive system as children, framing it instead as a specialised function with genetically determined machinery. By this thinking, it is not enough to be exposed to conversation, or else a puppy would pick up our language by hanging about the kitchen: we must have an innate capacity which allows us to combine linguistic elements into new structures that are more complex than anything we have been exposed to as we grow. Chomsky proposed the linguistic rules that allow us to do this, a universal grammar or 'language organ' evolved for that purpose, much as the motor or visual systems are specialised for their functions.

So what is happening as we turn the sound entering our ears into words, and from words into concepts, emotions or perhaps even poetry? The neurobiology of this language organ started gradually to come into focus only around the turn of this century as newer neuroscience techniques began to lift the lid on the language network. Auditory information from the ears first reaches the brain's cortex in Heschl's gyrus at the back of the temporal lobes on either side. This auditory cortex fires off when we process any sound and is not specific for language.

A crucial first step must be to discriminate sounds that are speech from those that are not and then to decode this into phonemes, the word fragments beloved of phonics teachers. Early acoustic analysis seems to take place in Heschl's gyrus and then the first discrimination of phonemes just in front of this in the superior temporal gyrus, the information working its way forwards as it is analysed. Injuries to this region cause pure 'word deafness', where written text can be understood but auditory comprehension is destroyed. Once we have identified the phonemes then the linguistic analysis can begin.

The German neuroscientist Angela Friederici has spent years chasing the path taken by a word or sentence as it makes its way through the brain and transforms from sound to sentence. She recorded and described an electrical waveform over frontal regions called Left Anterior Negativity which may reflect one of the earliest steps along this pathway, seen specifically in response to hearing an error of syntax known as a phrase structure violation. This may be triggered by a phrase such as 'my on bed' (instead 'on my bed') and is detected one or two hundred milliseconds after the sound.

Friederici and others have suggested a model in which sentence comprehension has three stages. First the structures of individual phrases are decoded – subject-verb-object, who is doing what to whom. Second, the structure of the sentence as a whole is determined, including semantic information (are the right kinds of words in the right places?) and how the phrases relate to each other syntactically. Finally there is some sort of integration whereby the overall meaning is extracted, around six hundred milliseconds after the sound. For a simple phrase – Anne kicks the ball – the overall meaning may be clear after the second stage. Interpreting a more complex sentence may depend on higher-level syntactic analysis or even on accessing contextual knowledge, thus taking longer.

This processing does largely seem to involve the network spanning the left temporal and frontal lobes, but dissecting out different types of task has revealed at least two separate streams of information flow. Parrot-fashion word repetition (including made-up words) involves a dorsal pathway from the superior temporal gyrus to the part of the inferior frontal gyrus considered Broca's area. A task that depends on comprehension, however, activates a more ventral pathway linking the temporal lobe to frontal regions tucked underneath and more laterally. This model creates a strong analogy with the visual system, with a dorsal stream that prepares a motor response and a ventral stream that extracts meaning. As always, though, the more you look the more you find. Functional brain imaging has now identified two dorsal and two ventral streams, each with distinct linguistic roles.

We now also know that while the bulk of semantic (extracting meaning) and syntactic processing is taking place in the brain's left hemisphere there are important roles being played also by the right. Prosody is the name given to the musical quality of speech, the variations in pitch and rhythm across a sentence that distinguish a monotone satnav voice from a stereotypical Welshman. Far from being an optional extra, prosody provides important information about meaning, clarifying boundaries between phrases and conveying emphasis. In many non-European languages tonal information is in fact essential to extract basic meaning. When trying to speak the coastal Ghanaian language Gã as a teen I found that the difference between a verb and its negative equivalent rested entirely on a subtle lengthening and upward inflexion of the key word. *Mi lé bo* for 'I know you' became *Mi lée bo* for 'I don't know you'. To my horror other variations in tone would change the verb's meaning completely. ('I would like to speak with your mother' held particular peril if mispronounced . . .)

Such tonal interpretation of syllables is probably part of the low-level acoustic analysis in Heschl's gyrus on the left side, but appreciating changes in pitch over seconds rather than milliseconds appears to involve equivalent regions on the right. Prosody has an essential role in conveying the emotional content of speech and this is recognised to depend on right-sided language regions. If you listen to a patient with a right-sided stroke talk, you often find that their speech has essentially normal content – no missing or jumbled words, correct grammar – but is oddly monotone and lacking in emotional punch.

In support of Chomsky's proposed hard-wired language organ, it seems that we are born with at least some of the wiring already functioning. It turns out that even pre-term babies at twenty-eight weeks gestation can discriminate a new syllable or a change in voice, detected as changes in blood flow in their frontal and temporal regions on both sides. Within five days of birth a baby's left temporal lobe responds specifically to speech, as opposed to the same sound played backward. Newborns can also 'learn' a new word within two minutes of hearing it, showing a greater blood flow response when hearing it again. By four months they can even discern the particular syllable stress patterns of their native language.

Attaching meanings to words – lexical knowledge – seems to take a little longer. As adults we show a 'mismatch response' in the form of an electrical deflection in the left hemisphere after hearing a word that does not match a picture we are looking at. Infants first develop this at around fourteen months. By the age of three a toddler will have grasped most of the rules of their native language and will know quite a few words. This coincides also with a recognised 'sensitive period' for language acquisition: a second language learnt before the age of three will usually be spoken indistinguishably from a native speaker, whereas after that age the same level of proficiency will rarely be reached.

But while an ankle-biter can get their meaning across, they do not speak in full, complex sentences, and this capacity does not usually mature until around the age of ten. This development coincides with a shift from a predominantly ventral stream of language processing to increasing use of the dorsal stream, and with maturation of the white matter tract linking the temporal and frontal lobes. This gives the language network access to heavy-duty processing power across our wider frontal networks, which can then get involved in complex sentences.

Some neuroscientists believe that development of this 'second dorsal stream' – weak in chimpanzees but strong in humans – was the key evolutionary step in humans that enabled complex language and so unleashed the cognitive revolution. This pathway may allow a more complex grammar whereby linguistic elements can be linked into infinite combinations by what Chomsky called the 'merge operation'. Wittgenstein famously declared that the limits of his language meant the limits of his world. If we believe that the evolution of complex language around thirty thousand years ago was synonymous with the emergence of full consciousness – the *Dust* of Philip Pullman's Lyra trilogy – then how this came about is an important and timely question. Each new iteration of artificial intelligence is based upon increasingly sophisticated versions of a 'large language model'. At present we have no idea what artificial 'evolutionary' step will transform such systems from linguistic party tricks into conscious entities with wills and agendas of their own. Nobody knows what the computational equivalent of a second dorsal stream would look like or if it is perhaps already underway. I confess that I do not look forward to finding out.

*

A few weeks after Dritan's arrival I walked into the day room to find the communication group in full swing. Laurel had gathered four of our patients around a large round wooden table in the corner near the games shelves. It was a crisp, clear morning and the table was caught in a shaft of bright but warmthless winter sun, which was doing little to melt the frost around the windows' edges. The activity in progress could perhaps be described as 'sitting around playing games and chatting' but in fact was more subtle and structured than appearances might suggest. Laurel was petite, with thick black hair cropped short and a small, high voice. She radiated kindness onto those around her like a benevolent sun and spirits were running high. Tarek was arranging Bananagram letters into fragments of rude words while two middle-aged men were playing Connect 4. They were watched by Terri, a recently admitted woman of seventy-odd with immaculately set blonde hair who, according to rumour, had been a music-hall singer back in the day.

Laurel was leading her group through a discussion of favourite singers. She carefully balanced her delivery according to the range of communication difficulties within the group, summarising back when it was unclear and gently drawing out those who found it harder. Terri had a Wernicke's aphasia – her most obvious difficulty was with comprehension, and while her speech was fluent the meaning was vague. Laurel wrote key words or made small drawings on a piece of paper as they went along, while the games served to take the pressure off the chat. The discussion turned to mainstream pop and it emerged that one of the Connect 4 players, a barrister in his late fifties, was a fanatical if slightly improbable Swiftie. Terri looked puzzled until Laurel wrote TAYLOR SWIFT in large letters and placed it before her. Terri frowned and cut in with a soft Yorkshire lilt.

'Oh no. No, no. You need to ginney. Ginney the rup. You find out the best and I like to, you see, I like to but not that one. Not that one. No that's all just whiney whiney girlie without any . . . without any real, you know, any real grut. The candom. You have to have a proper voicibubble to really do it, a good strong voicibubble with style not just . . . fluff! You need, you know . . . Frink. No, Frank.'

'Sinatra?' suggested Laurel.

Terri thumped the table in triumph. 'Absolutely!'

The barrister conceded the point graciously, though he continued quietly to make a rearguard case for Tay-Tay's wide range of vocal styles. At this point Tarek looked up from his game, pointed at the table and laughed out loud. The tiles spelled B-G-R-N-U-T-S. Laurel looked at him quizzically.

'Is that . . . buggernuts?'

Tarek threw his head back and roared. 'Yup, buggernuts!'

General laughter ensued and as it did the speech therapy assistant Helena hove into view up the ramp from the ward pushing Dritan in a chair. Laurel cleared a space for him around the table.

'Hello, Dritan. Welcome! How nice to see you!'

Helena set Dritan up with the noughts-and-crosses puzzle and he fiddled around with it while the discussion moved on to Ella Fitzgerald. Laurel tried a few times to bring him into the topic – we knew that he liked music and she suggested a number of singers he might appreciate – but he stared down at his puzzle and would not look up. After a few minutes he started to bang his left hand hard on the table. He then looked up, ground his teeth and swept the puzzle onto the floor. Helena took him back to his bay.

Dritan was not making progress and we were beginning to worry that the high level of stimulation he was receiving was serving only to increase his frustration. With no means of connecting with him, were our efforts perhaps making things worse?

Our music therapist Becky had her first session with Dritan that afternoon and by then he had settled back down. Laurel brought him into a small room tucked behind our reception and sat in to observe. This room was set up for music today, with a full-size keyboard in the middle and percussion instruments laid out along the worktop. Becky welcomed Dritan and introduced herself, then suggested they might play something together. Her smile conveyed a serene and entirely natural positivity – in her presence it was impossible but to believe that everything was going to be all right. She brought Dritan in line with the middle of the keyboard, sat to his left and began to play: a simple sequence of chords to start with, then adding a soft folky tune over the top with her voice. For a minute or so Dritan looked down at his lap and did nothing. As Becky left an expectant pause he looked up briefly. As she resumed playing he lifted his left hand to the keyboard and played a couple of tentative notes before snatching it quickly away. He groaned, gripped tightly on to his arm-rest and began to rock back and forth. Becky and Laurel tried to soothe Dritan but his groans only became louder and his rocking more violent. They had to abandon the session.

Later in the week Becky tried a different approach. This time it was just the two of them in the room and the keyboard was tucked away in the corner. Dritan seemed as sullen as last time and sat slumped in his wheelchair with his stare fixed on his lap.

Becky picked up an acoustic guitar and played a few chords. Dritan looked up, his ears visibly pricking. As Becky kept playing he leaned over towards her, so she held the guitar out, inviting him to strum while she held down the chords. It was 'Hey Jude' and he seemed to have no difficulty keeping the rhythm steady so she began to sing over the top and the song gathered momentum as they went. As they reached the 'La la la la-la-la lahs' Becky offered Dritan the neck of the guitar to see how he would respond. To her surprise, he started pressing down the rough chords as best he could with his left hand, leaving Becky to take over the strumming. At the final 'Hey Jude' she laughed and congratulated him. While he was not exactly smiling, he was sitting up straight and was entirely switched on. Dritan then caught sight of the keyboard in the corner: he looked up at Becky, raised his eyebrows and indicated it with his hand. They set themselves up and while she played chords at the bottom he improvised a tune over the top. His left hand was not as dexterous as you would expect of a regular pianist – this is often the case for the stronger hand in stroke, especially when there is apraxia – but he could manage perfectly well. The allotted time for the session's end came and went. Eventually another therapist needed the room and they had to stop, but Dritan had got the wind in his sails.

Listening to music really does make the brain light up like a Christmas tree. Imaging studies show activation in regions all across the brain, including cortical networks on both sides but also parts of the limbic system further down. This network mediates our emotional state and music provides a direct route into it which bypasses most higher cortical regions. So despite damage to movement, sensation or vision – even with loss of language, as in Dritan's case – music can induce the profoundest feelings and switch on activity across much of the brain. Music processing also stimulates parts of the right-sided language network – the same regions which interpret the prosody of speech – and boosting these may help to support recovering language function. Patients with aphasia who struggle to get words out can often sing pretty well, and this bypassing of left-sided damage can be harnessed. Melodic Intonation Therapy for aphasia involves attaching a simple tune to a short phrase with exaggerated melodic and rhythmic elements. This is repeated until it is learned and then the musical elements are gradually phased out, leaving a spoken phrase. But the most dramatic effect of music on our patients is on their mood and motivation, and Becky's group sessions are a core element of our unit's routine.

The following week Becky and Dritan were a few minutes into their session and were improvising a waltz on the keyboard when Sihana arrived on the ward. She found her brother's bed empty and a nurse indicated the music room, but when she heard the sounds emerging from within she did not for a moment think that this could be Dritan. She stuck her head around the corner of the door, saw Becky and Dritan playing and staggered back.

'But he's . . . How . . . ?'

Dritan looked over his shoulder, smiled at Sihana and continued to play. She was speechless. They had played duets growing up in Albania so she pulled up a chair and all three sat in a row at the keyboard: Becky continued with oompah-pahs at the bass end, while Sihana started to pick out chords in the middle and Dritan played a jaunty tune at the top. Then the siblings switched to a song that had the air of something from their childhood, and as Sihana accompanied her brother the tears ran down her cheeks.

Later that week Sihana brought her daughter Milla along, her reluctance to visit overcome by the news of this breakthrough. Milla sat in the corner of the little room while Dritan, Becky and Sihana worked their way through a song. As it finished with a flourish Dritan looked up at Milla with a broad grin, threw back his head and laughed.

*

Tarek had started to spend weekends at home, walking slowly by himself now with a high pole for support. We had suggested extending his admission by four weeks as he was clearly benefiting from the intensive speech therapy, and he reluctantly agreed. There were clear improvements. He was gradually enlarging the range of words that he could access, not all of them filthy, and was beginning to form simple phrases and short sentences. Laurel was drilling Tarek on re-training the link between pictures and words, putting phrases in the correct order and practising comprehension. She was also immersing him in groups, taking him to shops and setting up a video call with his family every afternoon, so that he could gain confidence implementing his training in real-world settings.

Tarek's pride and joy was a large red Kawasaki motorbike and, early on, he identified this as a word he wanted to be able to say. His word repetition was pretty good so Laurel started by getting him to repeat it back to her. She then removed one syllable at a time from her prompts, repeating this until Tarek could say the whole word from the truncated prompt before removing the next one: Ka-Wa-Sa-Ki, Ka-Wa-Sa, Ka-Wa, Ka. Finally, Tarek could say the word with no prompt at all. He was delighted.

For patients like Tarek it is likely that the problem is not so much his lexicon – the internal dictionary linking each object or concept to its word. Like episodic memory traces, words' actual representations are probably distributed widely across the brain's networks like a blockchain token – as such, they are hard to destroy in bulk. The issue is the mechanism of retrieving them, the fairground grabber, whose damage affects the ability to fish the words out. We all experience some retrieval difficulty at times, more so with ageing, familiar to many as 'tip-of-the-tongue' syndrome. When this happens we are aware that we have the word tucked away somewhere but cannot quite reach it. We can often recall the word's approximate shape as if we were seeing the outline of a figure through a blizzard. Sometimes mentally looking away helps it to pop back again. Word retrieval failure in aphasia is probably similar but on a grand scale.

We can now use functional imaging to see which brain regions are active during language use, and in a healthy person this is unsurprisingly the left language network. After a left-sided stroke causing aphasia a characteristic progression is typically seen. In the first few days the surviving brain regions around the stroke on the left are largely inactive, probably due to physical factors such as swelling. By twelve days some of these intact left-sided regions become active again but there is also extensive recruitment of language-equivalent regions on the right side, most strikingly in the right Broca's area. The extent of this rightward shift is greater in more severely affected patients. By one year post-stroke this activity has shifted to some extent back to the left side.

This shift to the opposite side after stroke has similarities to what we see for the control of movement, and just as for the motor system there is uncertainty as to whether this brain activity is doing anything helpful. We are in fact not entirely left-sided to start with: as children we use both sides to a degree and become progressively left-sided as we mature. There is some (admittedly mixed) evidence that women are less exclusively left-dominant than men, and left-handers of both sexes show a spectrum of left-versus-right language dominance. The language network has nodes on both sides and it seems to be capable of rapid plasticity, shifting its activity in response to change.

Intriguingly one such shift probably takes place when we learn to read. If we accept that writing in distinct characters first emerged around five thousand years ago, then literacy is not a capacity we have evolved to possess – natural selection has not had time to catch up, so the visual process of linking characters to sounds has been grafted onto a system designed to spot food and avoid predators. Imaging studies comparing illiterate adults to those who can read and to pre-readers suggest that a left-sided region specialised for facial recognition becomes 'recycled' for reading, somehow without a cost in facial recognition.

You can induce such shifts experimentally in healthy people. Researchers have used magnetic stimulation to suppress activity temporarily in the left inferior frontal gyrus (which includes Broca's area) – an effect lasting minutes – and then scanned with functional MRI to see which regions their subjects' brains were using to perform a language task. The activity in the stimulated region was reduced as expected but they also saw increased activation in other parts of the language network across both hemispheres and a stronger right-to-left connection between the two sides. This suggests that when it is disrupted the language network can rapidly redistribute computational power, remote regions taking up the slack from others when necessary.

Could the increased activity on the right side after stroke be propping up the struggling left language network? There is some support for this idea. When twenty patients with impaired word comprehension from a previous stroke were given intensive phonological training (matching sounds to words), they improved. No surprise there, perhaps, but subsequent brain imaging after training showed more language-related activity in their surviving left language regions and a stronger connection between the networks on each side.

Confusingly, though, this is not always the case. Several studies in aphasic patients have shown that inhibiting language regions on the right side with brain stimulation can be beneficial, suggesting the opposite conclusion. The timing after stroke is probably important: it may well be that early on, the right-sided hyperactivity results from a disturbed inhibitory balance between the two sides and is detrimental, whereas once the balance is re-established at a later stage the right side is able to lend support.

For now it remains unclear when or if to give brain stimulation for aphasia. For me, the key message from recent research is that the wider language network is capable of plasticity, engaging remaining language-capable regions in supporting communication, but that this depends on training and therapy. Interventions such as brain stimulation – when they are effective – are probably working by optimising the milieu for this neuroplasticity to take place. It also seems likely that the 'dose' of training is important in the extent of recovery, at least for patients with some remaining language regions. We now know that intensive therapy can bring about change even at a late stage. My colleagues Alex Leff and Jenny Crinion ran a study with forty-six aphasic patients who were an average of over two years down the road following stroke. Their patients received ninety hours of speech therapy over three weeks and saw significant and sustained improvements across all outcome measures. This result has been replicated a number of times elsewhere and the only reason such intensive programmes are not more common is the lack of available resources. As Alex put it, you would not treat a heart attack with just seven milligrams of aspirin.

*

It was the week before Tarek was due to go home and we were holding our Christmas party. Our redoubtable receptionist Nefertiti had been getting excited for weeks and had festooned the day room's walls with tinsel and colourful paperchains. Several of our staff had brought in food from home and the nurses had wrapped small presents for each of our patients, who sat gathered around tables with their families and the therapists. It was already dark outside and squalls of unseasonable rain lashed the windows on both sides, but somehow this served only to enhance the Christmas cheer and a happy hubbub permeated the large space.

Our rehab assistant Kevin had arranged a quiz and as he read out the questions in thick North London he made an unconventional Father Christmas, a red bobble hat perched on top of his shaved head. A senior colleague of mine used to dress up in full Santa gear every year, beard included, and would have his registrar follow him around the ward in an elf costume. Quite apart from the hallucinogenic effect such an apparition would have on a slightly confused patient (and the inevitable complaint from the junior doctor training committee), I had no desire to transform into a scary old man – I kept a low profile and banged out some carols on the keyboard while an assortment of the assembled company joined in and Becky accompanied on guitar. Laurel had tried to persuade Terri to sing a verse of 'Once in Royal David's City': she was not keen on this plan but did then launch unprompted into a stirring 'Danny Boy'. Allowing for the slight word salad resulting from her aphasia ('the peeps the peeps are bawling!') this was a real highlight and it was easy to imagine her holding the stage in years gone by.

Sihana sat with her husband and their children pulling crackers. Dritan remained largely mute but, since his music therapy sessions, he was a changed man. Something had clicked and he was now an enthusiastic participant in physio, walking around the ward unaided and even managing outside with a Nordic pole. He was also beginning to dress himself and was generally much less distressed. Sihana was very keen that he should not go back to his previous shared accommodation and wanted him to live near her family once he left hospital. They now planned to make him more a part of their life, so we were having complex discussions about sheltered accommodation with their local borough on the coast. Today Dritan was slowly making his way about the day room, a sparkly hat atop his head and a lop-sided gentle smile across his gaunt features, delivering to each table the slices of cake that Nefertiti was cutting.

I felt a tap on my shoulder. Tarek stood behind me with his wife looking on proudly. He held my arm and gathered himself.

'Doc, I want . . . I want to say. Your erm . . . your you know . . .' He paused and regrouped. 'Your team . . . amazing. Amazing! Laurel is really . . . she's . . .' He blew an extravagant kiss with his left hand. 'Mwooah!'

I thanked him – yes, the team were great.

'So, Tarek, seeing as you're so happy with your therapy how about we keep you here for another couple of months?'

He smiled. 'You must be . . . Fu . . . Fuck off, doc!'

CHAPTER TEN

THE HUNDRED-YEAR SULK

There was something going on in Saleh's brain but nobody was sure what it was. I took the call one Friday evening and the neurology registrar gave me the basics of the case. Saleh was in his twenties and previously well. He was Syrian and had moved to the UK around a year previously to live with his brother, Turki. Nine days ago Turki had taken Saleh to their local hospital's emergency department with concerns that he was behaving erratically. He had been vomiting that day and his symptoms were put down to a stomach bug, so he was sent home. Two days later Turki brought him back, as Saleh was now in a confused state. There was mention of possible drug use but few details.

The emergency department doctors had described Saleh as highly agitated, to the extent that security were keeping an eye on him. He was having frightening visual hallucinations, pointing at the walls and telling Turki that there were demons there who were trying to kill him. A physical examination revealed a confused man but was otherwise unrevealing; routine blood tests were normal and a plain CT brain scan showed nothing untoward. The nurses dipped his urine and found traces of cocaine: Turki admitted that Saleh had recently begun to use drugs, much to his despair as an older brother. He had never shown any signs of mental illness before and, in the context, a drug-induced psychosis was diagnosed. Psychiatry placed Saleh under section and transferred him to a local mental health centre for observation and treatment with anti-psychotic medication.

While there, however, he deteriorated. First he became yet more confused, unsure even of which country he was in, then he stopped speaking altogether. His limbs gradually stiffened and soon he was unable to walk or to eat. On the third day, the nurses found Saleh unresponsive and foaming from the mouth, so they sent him back to the emergency department. The doctors noted that he was semi-catatonic, not responding or speaking, and that his arms and legs seemed rigid. The presence of a cut inside his mouth also suggested uncontrolled jaw clenching, often the hallmark of an epileptic seizure.

This time the scan was not normal. There was patchy darkness in the brain's white matter on both sides, pretty extensive and certainly new since three days previously. There were several possible causes for this appearance – infection and inflammation were top of the list – but all that could be said at this point was that Saleh had some sort of widespread white matter abnormality. Before any more scans or tests could be done, he had a full-blown epileptic seizure and needed sedation and intubation in that hospital's ICU. Would we accept him as a transfer to our hospital for investigation?

Having started as a psychiatry case, Saleh now fell squarely within the remit of neurology. He was transferred that night and I saw him in the morning with the registrar and our ICU team. We gave him a thorough going-over and found stiffness in his limbs as described, but also brisker reflexes than normal: this usually suggests there is damage to the brain's pathways controlling movement, not surprising given the scan. We examined Saleh's body carefully for clues as to what could be causing this – skin, nails, joints, heart and the rest – but nothing jumped out. We began arranging tests.

Saleh's brother Turki had followed him to our ICU and he waited nervously outside while we did our thing. Once we were finished, we took him to the unit's quiet room to get some more background and he was very forthcoming.

'First I would like to say Saleh is not a bad boy. Always at home he was the good one, dutiful with our parents and good in his studies. But since coming to this country . . . it's been hard for him.'

I reassured Turki that nobody was judging his brother – we just needed to know more about him in order to give him the right treatment. I told him that we had found dark patches on Saleh's brain scan and were arranging tests but, at the moment, we did not know what these changes were. Anything he could tell us might be useful. Turki closed his eyes for a few seconds then leaned wearily back in the soft chair, the fluorescent ceiling lights picking him out with an oddly two-dimensional quality.

Saleh was one of several children in their family, he told us, and had been the golden boy, clever in school and the apple of their father's eye. As the war in Syria tore their life apart Saleh was picked up at a checkpoint because one of his brothers had attended a protest march. He wound up in one of Assad's prisons, where he was tortured, but eventually the goons lost interest and turned him out. He managed to flee the country and made it to Holland, where he spent three years before gaining entry to the UK to join Turki. All was well at first and Saleh had enrolled in an electrical engineering course. Some months ago, though, he had begun to drink too much and then got in with a bad crowd locally. Much as Turki had pleaded with him, he had stopped turning up to college and often smelled of weed. Turki shood his head sadly.

'In Syria he saw too many bad things. Too many.'

On the night Saleh was admitted to hospital Turki had gone looking for him, wandering around the darker corners of their neighbourhood. He followed the canal's towpath away from the main road and was about to give up when he came across Saleh under a bridge, crouched in the shadows beyond the harsh yellow light of the sodium lamps. He was holding some sort of pipe with a bag of white powder and seemed scared, talking to himself. Turki was furious and threw the drug paraphernalia into the canal. He did not know for sure what it was but guessed cocaine.

This account made sense of the urine dip result but did not on its own explain what we were seeing. Cocaine in large doses can certainly cause strokes or bleeds but not the sort of brain-wide changes that we could see on Saleh's scan, nor the gradually worsening clinical course he had followed. We found no specific clues from his spinal fluid nor from a long list of blood tests. We got him into an MRI scanner and this gave us a much clearer view of the changes on both sides. They were very widespread and resembled either severe inflammation – an autoimmune condition known as ADEM – or widespread chemical toxicity of some kind. Of these, ADEM has a specific treatment, so we gave Saleh high-dose steroids and filtered antibodies out of his bloodstream for five days.

One of our registrars meanwhile did some digging into cocaine contaminants: there were batches circulating London then in which the drug had been cut with an anti-worming powder used in cattle. This could cause toxic reactions in humans, and there were a few reports of patchy white matter changes in the brain. This seemed like a good lead but we needed some evidence and the original sample was at the bottom of a canal. By now this substance would have been metabolised so blood tests would not be helpful. We could take a biopsy from an affected region of his brain but this is clearly very invasive and would come with risks. So we cut off a chunk of his armpit hair (the longest hair we could find) and sent it to a helpful professor in Paris whose lab could perform the test. He emailed me the following week: the hair contained high levels of this anti-worming drug.

By now Saleh was beginning to improve – ICU had been able to remove the tube from his airway and had begun to wake him up. We stopped the steroids, which would most likely not help, treated him for seizures and let time take its course. He was groggy to start with but once he was moved to a medical ward he began to surface and was able to shuffle about and speak a little. Bit by bit he could tell us where he was and what had happened. He was no longer hallucinating but was still quite paranoid – he thought that his phone was listening in on him (to be fair he may have a point) and, when I visited, he paced about his room like a caged leopard, peering around with a hunted look. At one point, as his distress mounted he started to bang his head against the wall so we asked a mental health nurse to sit with him and again involved psychiatry. Though he was slowly improving, Saleh was too mentally disturbed to manage in the highly stimulating environment of our rehabilitation unit, so we referred him to a psychiatry-led neurobehavioural centre.

Saleh's medical care had moved between psychiatry and neurology as his dominant symptoms had shifted between mental and physical manifestations of brain dysfunction. If somebody has a pure disturbance of their mental state then their care falls under psychiatry. The moment there is an abnormal physical finding – a fever, or an abnormal movement – or something is found on a brain scan, then their case is deemed neurological.

*

The most common transient disturbance of mental function (if you except booze) is delirium, a confusion of mind which may be hyperactive and agitated in the young but in the elderly often produces an almost catatonic state of inactivity. The brain usually appears normal on scanning but there is a metabolic disturbance compromising its function – commonly infection, though not always – and as this resolves the fog clears. The symptoms can include hallucinations or delusional beliefs – the nurses are trying to kill me! – and yet this is not considered psychiatric, being a mental manifestation of a physical disturbance. While in northern Ghana some years ago I lay in a hospital bed with a high fever from bacterial dysentery (if I had been designing the hospital I would probably have put the toilets in the same block as the ward – just saying). In the middle of the night an insect in the bushes of the hospital garden started up with an intermittent high-pitched sound, a short ping every few seconds that was probably not that loud but which reverberated like a bell inside my head. In my febrile state I became firmly convinced that this sound was my heart monitor – it was running dangerously slowly, was nobody going to do anything? – and worked myself into quite a froth about it. My long-suffering friend was dozing in a chair by the bed. He pointed out that there was no monitoring equipment.

Delirium often waxes and wanes before it clears up completely but can sometimes go on for days. Some months before her eventual demise, our family friend Jenny was admitted to her local hospital with a chest infection. She was as sharp as anybody and with a rapier wit to boot, but with the infection her oxygen levels dropped and her temperature rose, sending her into a drowsy and confused state. A week later she rallied spectacularly and was soon back to her excellent self. Her son had been watching over her and asked whether she had been aware of being perilously ill.

'Every night as I lay here,' she told him, 'Death came to visit. He sat on the end of my bed and talked to me for hours.'

Slightly perturbed, her son asked what Death had been like.

'He was a crashing bore. After a few nights of this I had had enough so I told him to fuck off. I never saw him again.'

We often see psychiatric consequences in conditions that are clearly neurological but whose effects include changes in mental processes. The core symptoms of Parkinson's disease are tremor, stiffness and slow movement due to declining dopamine levels within the brain. Almost half of patients with this condition have depressive symptoms which can develop years before the physical symptoms emerge, probably because of declining levels of serotonin and other neurotransmitters. Later on many also experience characteristic visual hallucinations. An array of psychiatric symptoms are likewise seen in Huntington's disease – a genetically determined degenerative condition whose most obvious manifestation is a dance-like movement known as chorea – and in encephalitis, as Priya had experienced.

These are neurological conditions which disturb function across much or even all of the brain – it would be odd if they did not have some effect on mental processes – but we see mental health symptoms also with more localised damage. Somewhere around a third of patients with stroke will go on to have a significant depressive episode during their recovery, most then resolving after a year or more. Sometimes patients' sadness may simply reflect an appropriate response to a crappy turn of events, what psychiatrists call an adjustment disorder. Often, though, it appears to be more than this. Patients with stroke have far more depressive symptoms than those similarly incapacitated for other reasons, for example after orthopaedic injuries. Metabolites of serotonin within the spinal fluid are depleted in post-stroke depression, and different aspects of the overall depressive syndrome – poor motivation, impaired concentration, anxiety, sadness – can be related to damage in specific regions.

These strands of evidence suggest there may be a biological process by which stroke can induce a depressive state, and one theory is that the cerebral cortex is lacking monoamines. These are a group of neurotransmitters which modulate synaptic transmission within the cerebral cortex. Their effects are legion but the states they promote can perhaps be summarised as happiness for serotonin, arousal for noradrenaline and reward and satisfaction for dopamine. These monamines are synthesised down in the brainstem, from where a pathway for each projects upwards and distributes their powerful effects across the brain's hemispheres from below, like neural sprinklers of motivation and drive. A stroke may interrupt these projections and deplete the cortex of monoamines.

*

Patricia was a catering assistant from Essex in her fifties who suffered a stroke obstructing her basilar artery, a large vessel which sits in front of the brainstem and supplies much of the blood to the base and back of the brain. The obstruction was only partial and the clot was fished out by a radiologist – complete basilar obstruction is often fatal – but she sustained damage to many brain regions, including parts of her brainstem, temporal and occipital lobes. Patricia had profound weakness of her right arm and leg but also visual field loss and hemispatial neglect on that side. She came to us some months later, having had a number of medical issues along the way, and on arrival was in a poor state. Apart from her neurological impairments the main issue was a high level of distress, often crying inconsolably from a combination of physical discomfort and the position in which she found herself.

At the height of Patricia's distress she began to hallucinate, seeing members of her family or strangers in her room when there were none. She had a bladder infection at the time which was likely a factor, and her condition improved when we treated this, but while the visions settled she remained convinced that there was a baby somewhere in the room. At times she could hear it crying. Gradually this baby then took up residence in

Patricia's right arm. Since arrival she had struggled to identify this limb as her own: when the physios asked her to point out her right arm she could not find it, irritably scooping it out of the way with her left hand and digging around in the bedclothes beneath it. When they showed it to her, she could not say whose it was. They identified her shoulder for her, which Patricia acknowledged as her own, and then worked their way down the limb until she reluctantly admitted it was hers. She started referring to a baby in her bed and when asked where it was would indicate her right arm. She told us that the baby was not moving because it was weak – she needed to feed it. At one point she thought the baby had died and became inconsolable, though fortunately it revived before too long.

Patricia had formed a delusional system out of a distorted sensory and perceptual field – a situation pompously named somatoparaphrenia, which is probably an extension of neglect. It may be that the sensory information from the arm never reaches higher cortical regions and so cannot complete the feedback loop back down to the limbic system. This usually confers a sense of familiarity with the limb: lacking this hit, the brain concludes that it must belong to somebody else.

Around that time we also took on Mirdhu, a woman in her early sixties who with her husband had moved to the UK from Sri Lanka in the late 1980s, like many others fleeing the civil war there. Mirdhu had suffered an intracranial bleed which left her with profound weakness on her right side but also with severely slurred speech due to tongue weakness, such that she needed to point to a chart for communication.

Mirdhu was suspicious of staff members, accusing nurses of tampering with her food and insisting on the curtains around her bed always being drawn. And while her husband seemed nice enough at a superficial level, in sessions with our neuropsychologist Mirdhu began to paint a different picture. She told us that he had taken funds out of their import business for himself, that he stole money from her at home and was sometimes physically abusive. This claim necessarily triggered a safeguarding alert and he was confined to supervised visits until we could dig further. Our safeguarding team could not find any evidence of abusive behaviour on her husband's part, though of course you can never be certain. Most oddly, perhaps, Mirdhu was also entirely convinced that her husband had secretly replaced her children with impostors three years previously – her son and daughter were lookalike stand-ins that he had arranged.

We spoke to several members of Mirdhu's family, including her children, and a picture emerged of mental health difficulties going back some time. She had always been an anxious person but had changed dramatically following her first stroke three years earlier, a right parietal bleed which extended downwards to involve lower regions. The physical symptoms had largely resolved, but overnight she had become highly suspicious of everyone and everything. It was then that she first mentioned her suspicions that her children had been switched: they had muddled through, but with the new stroke everything was amplified.

This delusional belief about her children's identities is known as Capgras syndrome, after the doctor who first described it, and is usually seen in the context of psychotic conditions such as schizophrenia or in some forms of dementia. In Mirdhu's case, this belief was not isolated but was part of a wider array of psychiatric symptoms. Nonetheless the location of her stroke fitted into a model in which there is disconnection between facial recognition and the emotional processing that would usually accompany it.

The process of decoding an image into a familiar face takes place in the fusiform gyrus, a region tucked under the temporal lobes. This is linked by white matter tracts to distant regions for further processing, including the limbic system, which generates an emotional response to the face in question. In Capgras syndrome, so the theory goes, the patient consciously recognises the face and yet does not receive the emotional hit from it that they would expect. The brain does not like cognitive dissonance, so it draws the only logical conclusion: the person must be an impostor. It took a careful mix of neuropsychology, psychiatry and mental health-trained nursing to get Mirdhu gradually into a state where she began to trust the team and make progress.

*

The division of neurology from psychiatry as separate disciplines is something of a historical accident, emerging out of dramatically different directions taken by key nineteenth-century figures. The year 2025 marked the two hundredth anniversary of the birth of Jean-Martin Charcot, the bombastic Parisian physician who looms over Victorian medicine and who is generally regarded as the father of neurology as a speciality. There is almost no branch of medicine to which Charcot did not in some way contribute, and he achieved a previously unheard-of degree of status and fame. The Salpêtrière hospital in Paris sits near the banks of the Seine and had been first an armaments factory under Louis XIII, then a women's prison and subsequently an alms house. After the revolution it evolved into an asylum and hospital and hosted a number of legendary physicians, but under Charcot's stewardship it achieved international renown as a centre of neurology. There, he supposedly took personal charge of up to three thousand inpatients at a time.

Charcot was a great believer in localising the site of the pathology underlying a disorder. His technique of correlating autopsy findings with patients' symptoms and examination findings led ultimately to the clinical method that still underpins neurology practice. He would give dramatic demonstrations of his method at the Salpêtrière, watched by admiring physicians who would travel from afar to be present. The most notorious of these was captured on canvas by André Brouillet and depicts one of Charcot's most celebrated patients, known as Blanche, in a dramatic swoon while the master physician, turning away from the patient, addresses his audience of stolid frock-coated men. This was a demonstration of hysteria, a state of incapacity or seizure-like movements induced in these sessions by hypnosis or by physical pressure over the abdomen. Charcot mistakenly attributed these symptoms, which might now be described as psychosomatic, to transient swelling of the brain.

Watching one of Charcot's demonstrations was a young Sigmund Freud. In considering the basis of hysteria he was greatly influenced by the writings of Pierre Janet, another of Charcot's disciples, who proposed an important role for the subconscious (a term that Freud coined in 1893) in generating hysterical symptoms. Along with fellow Viennese Josef Breuer, Freud developed this idea into a fully formed theory in their controversial book *Studies on Hysteria*, which suggested that hysterical symptoms were manifestations of historical traumatic experiences bubbling up from the subconscious and taking on physical form. Freud rejected what he saw as the increasing obsession with localising physical lesions in the brain in favour of a model in which subconscious mental processes surface and may overwhelm conscious behaviour. This led, ultimately, to *The Interpretation of Dreams* and what became known as the talking cure. Psychoanalysis was born.

In the late nineteenth century these two competing philosophies of the brain's dominion over the body rapidly diverged. The practice of localising lesions in the brain was going from strength to strength, championed by the giant figure of Charcot. Set against this was the burgeoning field of psychoanalysis, swept along by Freud and his disciples, which sought to use an entirely different approach to explain not just mental disorders but many apparently physical manifestations too. This schism became entrenched as the respective fields of psychiatry and neurology developed their own trainings, cultures and methodologies. It has persisted for over a century.

For an example of how this divergence of approaches has been less than productive one might consider the childhood onset tic disorder Tourette syndrome, which has bounced for over a hundred years between the two fields. The condition is associated in the popular imagination with involuntary swearing – coprolalia – though in fact the vocal tics can take a variety of forms. Even now its cause remains poorly understood but it is generally viewed as a neurodevelopmental disorder and has associations with learning difficulty and attention deficit. However, a high proportion of its sufferers also show obsessive-compulsive behaviours and other symptoms that would fall squarely into the field of psychiatry. Gilles de la Tourette himself was yet another of Charcot's acolytes (you can even see him in Brouillet's painting, sitting in the front row) and considered his patients to have a form of hereditary insanity, distinguished from hysteria by their inability to 'cure' it using hypnosis. Meanwhile Freud and his supporters considered the condition a variety of hysteria resulting from subconscious inner struggles and sexual repression, and the vocal tics a symbolic expression of masturbation. As recently as the 1985 Paris symposium marking the centenary of the condition's description there is said to have been fierce and acrimonious division between camps arguing for a strictly 'organic' (meaning physical) basis and those insisting on a strict psychodynamic explanation – American versus French respectively.

The more light that neuroscience has shed on such conditions – and on the workings of the brain in general – the less sense it makes to maintain such a strict separation between neurology and psychiatry. The eminent American neurologist Stanley Cobb made an early attempt to bring the two disciplines closer together. Arriving at Harvard as an epilepsy neurologist in the 1930s he adopted psychiatric methods including psychoanalysis (he is even said to have personally shone the shoes of Carl Jung while putting him up for the night) and championed the concept of neuropsychiatry. Regarding the disciplinary schism he wrote: 'There is no biological significance to this division; it is simply an administrative affair, so that the university president will know what salary goes to which professor.'

With the development of more sophisticated research methods, the neuroscience on which the two clinical disciplines lean has steadily converged, revealing beyond doubt that biological changes are seen in psychiatric conditions, such as changes in frontal lobe activation in depression. The advent of drugs which treat psychiatric conditions by altering brain chemistry – anti-psychotics which reduce dopamine, anti-depressants which increase serotonin – have been further steps towards a more biological perspective on mental illness. It is important to emphasise that the existence of biological changes in mental health disorders does not by any means reduce the importance of psychological factors, nor of talking-based treatments. As people we are products not only of our biology but of the experiences we accumulate throughout life and of our social contexts: to ignore the role these factors play would be as foolhardy as to deny the influence of biology on psychiatry.

The separation of training resulting from the historical parting of ways has made us neurologists poor at detecting mental health issues when they arise. But more than a century after these two disciplines parted ways – not always on the best of terms – we have more recently seen a reconvergence of approach. By 1994 an editorial in the journal *Neurology* declared 'Neuropsychiatry is foreseeably on a growth trajectory'. Neuropsychiatry has become an integral part of our rehabilitation team and my only reflection now is to wonder how we managed previously.

It is increasingly clear that intention and thought cannot be separated from the brain's physiological and biochemical processes, nor from its anatomy. Equally the physical functions of our nervous systems cannot be separated from our mental processes, many of which may be subconscious. A view has emerged in which the brain and the mind are two co-dependent aspects of the same entity, the border between which, if it exists at all, is fluid and permeable. If this is true, then how the machineries of movement or perception function at any given moment must be subject to the ebb and flow of our mental processes.

*

Lee joined us one summer afternoon and was in a sorry state. Tall, lean and pale as a full moon, he was in his early twenties, raised in a tough London neighbourhood that politics had forgotten. I knew little of his personal history when he arrived but there was a sense that his upbringing had not been easy. He was brittle in his interactions, defensive with doctors and bore literal scars from his childhood. There was a small loyalty tattoo on his left wrist and he had told physios at the previous hospital that he was involved in a local gang. During the spring Lee had begun to feel a burning sensation in his feet as if he had scalded them in a hot bath. This feeling spread over a week or so to his knees and then to his hands. It was painful enough to need painkillers and for a while he soldiered on, but soon he started to feel wobbly on his feet. Within four weeks he was unable to walk and took to his bed.

By the time Lee was admitted to his local hospital he was in severe pain, requiring morphine, and could not sit up without help. His vision was blurry. When the doctors examined him his limbs were extremely sensitive to touch: he shouted out with any contact and kept the bedclothes off his feet. As well as pain there was a loss of sensation to touch and temperature in his hands and feet. They found that the usual reflexes in his arms and legs were absent, suggesting a problem with his nerves, and this was confirmed with electrical testing.

The most common cause for a rapid loss of nerve function is an inflammatory condition called Guillain-Barré syndrome, often seen weeks or days after an infection of some kind, in which our immune system makes antibodies that attack and strip the myelin sheaths off our nerves. Lee was treated for this with infusions of pooled antibodies called immunoglobulin, but he did not improve, and once a neurologist had assessed him they felt this was not the cause of his problems. They noted that he had a poor diet and asked him questions about drug use. Other than the occasional bit of weed, Lee denied taking anything strong – certainly no cocaine or similar. The neurologist asked him specifically about nitrous oxide, a brief buzz-giver often inhaled at parties from little metal cylinders, and he admitted that he was partial to this. In fact around the time his symptoms had started he had been on a bit of a splurge, on one occasion getting through two boxes in one night. Each box contained twenty-five cylinders. The neurologist arranged some specialist blood tests and confirmed the diagnosis: neuropathy due to severe nutritional deficiency.

Many people run slight deficiencies of vitamins, most commonly vitamin D from a lack of sun exposure – the endless grey lid under which we live. Diets such as veganism or just poor general nutrition often lead to a lack of the B vitamins and this can affect nerve function. A deficiency in thiamine, for example, can compromise the brain and particularly in alcoholics can lead to a confused state or even severe and permanent memory loss. A lack of B12 or riboflavin tends to damage the peripheral nerves in the limbs and some of the tracts in the spinal cord. If the levels are low but the nerves are just about managing then nitrous oxide can tip them over the edge, inactivating any B12 that is around and precipitating a metabolic crisis. The clues in Lee's case had been the severe pain at the time of onset and a hunch about his diet. The treatment is an aggressive replacement of vitamins in high doses, but often the nerves have taken a significant hit by that time. Since the UK's welfare state was hollowed out by government after the 2008 financial crisis this condition has been seen increasingly frequently – I would now describe it as common.

When Lee moved to our ward I went to meet him at the bedside. Bay 4 was still closed for refurbishment (I made a mental note to find out what was going on in there) and his bed was further down the ward, opposite two middle-aged men with strokes. Lee was rather surly with me to start with but he warmed up as we went along, and peeping out from behind the studied nonchalance were flashes of warmth and humour. He had the blue curtain pulled closed around his bedspace and had been listening to drill music on his phone when I came in. He turned it off and I helped him up onto the edge of the bed. His dark tracksuit bottoms and hoodie hung loosely from his long frame like paper on a saggy kite.

Examining him, I found subtle thinning of the muscles in his feet but only mild weakness in his legs. When I tried to elicit reflexes with a tendon hammer these were not there. The most striking findings, however, were abnormalities of sensation. He flinched from pain whenever I touched his feet and when I applied vibration to bony prominences (using a large tuning fork) he could not feel this at all below his ankles or wrists. I asked him to close his eyes and his fingers and arms drifted about as if untethered. When I moved his toes up or down he could not tell me which way they were going.

As I lifted up Lee's T-shirt to examine his torso I had a surprise. Running in parallel down his back was a series of thick pale pink lines, a foot or more long in places and shiny against his milk-white skin. He heard my involuntary intake of breath and met my eye.

'Do you mind if I ask how you got these, Lee?'

He shrugged. 'When I was younger I lived with my uncle for a while. He had a cat-o'-nine-tails. It's OK. He's nothing.'

This really was not nothing and for a while I froze. From Lee I could feel a little pride in these war wounds which he had survived but also the sadness that surrounded how he came by them. I felt like a physician in the London of Dickens – yet here we were in the twenty-first century. I asked Lee a little more about his diet. He ate a lot of chicken wraps and told me that he was not a fan of veg. I asked if he had any greens at all. He grinned.

'I had a bit of broccoli once when I was about ten. Never again.'

Once the physios started to get Lee into the gym and on his feet they found the going pretty hard. They stood him up between three therapists to start with but as he tried to maintain an upright posture his legs wobbled from side to side like early Elvis. If he closed his eyes it was dramatically worse – lacking the usual sensation, he was relying more on visual feedback. When he tried to take steps with a frame his legs would jerk violently and unpredictably. These movements could be attributed at least in part to a loss of sensation but gradually it seemed that this was not the only issue at play. Sometimes his legs gave jerks even when he was sitting resting. During sessions his arms would suddenly shake from side to side as if somebody were playing with a rag doll – this might continue for a few minutes and then stop. When it happened the therapists found that if they distracted Lee then the jerks subsided. These movements often started in the run-up to a difficult task in therapy.

The question we began to ask ourselves was whether some of Lee's symptoms might have a psychosomatic basis. Such symptoms are often now termed 'functional', meaning a disturbance of how the system is functioning, but confusing terminology abounds. The word 'psychogenic' is often used, and such patients may also be described as having a conversion disorder. If Charcot were in our gym (which, oddly enough, he probably was when he visited in the 1880s and watched Victor Horsley perform early neurosurgery) he would call this hysteria.

While we were wondering about this Lee developed a new symptom: he was in bed and about to be taken for therapy when he closed his eyes, sank back and started shaking all four limbs. His arms and legs were floppy and his head moved from side to side. This had all the hallmarks of a non-epileptic seizure, also known as dissociation, a further functional symptom in which a patient loses control of their body for a period of time. We arranged an electrical test of his brain waves to reassure ourselves that we were not wrong and, as expected, this was normal. With respect to the possible functional limb movements this development was something of a clincher.

Functional symptoms are not in any sense deliberate in that they are beyond conscious control. They are also just as 'real' as other symptoms, and patients who suffer from them wish that they would stop. Lee had severe nerve damage onto which these additional symptoms were layered, and it is often the case that functional and organic (or physical) symptoms coexist. The functional symptoms – whether jerks, apparent paralysis or seizure-like episodes – can be thought of as an abnormality of how the body's machinery is being used rather than a defect in the machinery itself. The computing analogy is useful here and neurologists will often explain such symptoms to patients in terms of a software issue: the hardware is intact but is receiving the wrong instructions. Another useful perspective is to consider that the brain has learned an incorrect movement pattern. Anybody who has learned to play a piece of music knows that sometimes you get stuck on one particular passage. Having played it wrong a few times the mistake becomes entrenched and then every time you get to that bar it comes out jumbled (or maybe it is just the way I practise). Once this has happened it is hard to unlearn it but crucially it is not impossible: you can re-train your fingers into the right pattern.

The origin of functional symptoms has been much debated. Freud framed them in terms of repressed desires or unprocessed early trauma breaking out of the subconscious. If you go looking for previous trauma or mental health symptoms then you will find them in a greater proportion of people who have functional symptoms than in those who do not – it would seem foolhardy to dismiss Lee's run-ins with the cat-o'-nine-tails from somehow being relevant – but there are plenty of patients with functional symptoms and no such history. The issue presumably lies somewhere at the brain–mind interface. Even the word *psycho-somatic* means 'of the mind and of the body', or perhaps the conscious experiencing of the body. One can imagine mental processes leeching across into the realm of motor control and disrupting its processes. But how?

The best current theory, in my view, sees functional symptoms as a disruption of the internal models by which we control and interpret our environment. We are familiar with this in our cerebellum's smoothing-out of reaching movements – making feed-forward predictions of the results of a command to move, then adjusting the model if it is inaccurate. It is likely that our brains employ such a modelling approach more widely. In this view the brain is not a passive regurgitator, automatically processing stimuli and churning out responses, but an organ that is actively seeking to solve the maths problem of the world we inhabit, making sense of it according to what it expects to find. Pioneering English neuropsychiatrist Michael Trimble called this the 'intentional brain'.

A model which makes predictions using probabilities that change as evidence accumulates is referred to as Bayesian, after the branch of statistics on which it is based. Searching for your glasses in the house, the probability of finding them in a given room increases with every room that you eliminate. This is an efficient way to incorporate uncertainty into predictions, so Bayesian modelling seems well suited to the brain as it handles a messy and uncertain world.

Another way to think of such a system is that it is comparing bottom-up sensory evidence with top-down predictions and calculating a prediction error from the difference between them. The top-down prediction is based upon a prior belief – what sensory feedback would the model 'expect' to result from a given movement? Once a comparison is made with the actual feedback received then the resulting prediction error updates the model. By gradually minimising this error, the prior belief is optimised until the model works well.

According to this theory of functional symptoms the problem starts when the person in question for some reason develops either an abnormal prior belief or a distortion of sensory input, and consequently experiences an unusually large prediction error. This will be familiar to anybody who has stepped onto a broken escalator: at a conscious level we know we will not feel the usual jolt and yet somehow there is still a disconcerting adjustment – a mismatch between what our model expects and what it receives – which makes us feel transiently unsteady. In Lee's case the abnormal sensory input may be the result of his damaged nerves, but in some patients the trigger could be something as innocuous as a minor injury, like a sprained ankle.

Faced with a large prediction error the brain usually just updates the model and moves on, but in patients with functional symptoms this does not happen and it becomes entrenched. This is a result of the second key ingredient, according to this theory: a pathologically exaggerated attentional focus on sensory errors.

At some level we all recognise the detrimental effect of excessive attention. If while walking down the street we start to think too much about which foot goes in front of which then our normal patterns start to break down and we almost trip. We have all seen top-level tennis players whose serve falls to pieces as the pressure of 'the mental game' focuses excessive attention on what is usually to them an automatic movement. It is easy to imagine how somebody's mental state could influence how they direct their attention or how prior traumatic experiences could play a role.

Attempting to resolve this exaggerated mismatch drives the system to adjust sensations or even make movements to align the bottom-up feedback with the expectation from the prior belief and so minimise the error. Crucially, because these adjustments are not generated at the conscious top end of the hierarchy – and the feedback resulting from them may be different from what was predicted – they may feel involuntary. This 'misattribution of agency' makes the movements generated by the abnormally functioning system feel beyond the patient's conscious control.

This model also allows for local belief systems or expectations to influence how symptoms develop. The prevalence of whiplash – neck discomfort persisting for months after a relatively minor rear-end driving collision – varies enormously between countries. It is almost unheard of in Greece, for example, but very common in Canada, despite no significant difference in accidents. There is, however, a large difference in expectations between the two countries as to what sort of symptoms people might expect after a minor collision: in countries where whiplash is not expected it simply does not exist.

For therapists treating patients with functional symptoms this model has important practical implications. If excessive focus on movements and sensations is part of the problem then moving the spotlight away from what the patient is doing should help. Distracting attention away from the action in progress turns down the gain on sensory mismatches and allows more normal movement patterns to be gradually restored. Once the physios began to do this with Lee, introducing deliberate distraction techniques to their sessions, he started to make progress with walking. Once he was more settled on the ward and less rattled by what the therapists were trying to do with him, the seizure-like episodes stopped entirely.

For Lee the functional limb jerks were only part of what he was having to deal with, and even with these eliminated the loss of feedback from his limbs made smooth movement difficult. Once the cores of the peripheral nerves are damaged – the axons themselves rather than just the myelin sheaths around them – they take a long time to recover, regrowing from the spinal cord by around a millimetre each day. From the lumbar spine to the feet may be a metre or more in some people – that is between two and three years of growth. Unlike the brain, there is no capacity for networks to reorganise – it is essentially a cable issue – so therapy concentrates on making the most of what function there is, preventing any secondary problems developing in the soft tissues and teaching compensatory techniques to achieve basic tasks. Lee was able to look after himself with only minor help within a few weeks but independent mobility was going to take much longer, and he would still need a wheelchair by the time he left us. Not easy for anybody but particularly perhaps for him, with a complicated home situation and shaky support networks.

At the end of Thursday afternoons our music therapist Becky would set up the gym for a music group and I found Lee there one day with two members of his family. He took this group extremely seriously and had insisted that they not only come along but also join in, so the three of them sat with four or so other patients and filled the large space with riotous music. Becky was leading the session from the keyboard in theory but

I could see that the song they were performing had taken on a life of its own.

Juliette was a smartly dressed and rather severe woman in her sixties who before a recent stroke had practised as a barrister specialising in international shipping. I could well imagine her in a wig and gown but today she had requested 'What Shall We Do with the Drunken Sailor?' and was making a determined effort to get through all the verses. Patricia had joined in with a lively tambourine (the mysterious baby now quite forgotten) and Becky accompanied on keyboard. At some point Lee had gone off script, adding a few improvisations here and there to start with but then moving into a full rap. Not to be discouraged, Juliette carried doggedly on with the song and as she caught Lee's eye they exchanged mischievous smiles. The drill-sea-shanty picked up and Lee's rap became more animated, something about 'My girl Julie' sorting your boats out. As the tempo increased our rehab assistant Comfort added a Nigerian dance, bottom low to the ground and arms raised, and by now Becky was having hysterics. I left them to it.

CHAPTER ELEVEN

THE MURKY DEPTHS

I was working my way around the wards of a district general hospital, reviewing patients who had been referred for a neurology opinion. There had been ten or so referrals for that afternoon so far, and I had about three hours to see them, so even supported by a junior doctor I was having to set a briskish pace. Most were pretty straightforward – adjusting epilepsy medications, Parkinson's disease, bad headaches – and it was possible to make a swift clinical decision and move on. If there was an unclear diagnosis, however, or something potentially serious then these consultations could take considerably longer. That day I had nipped into the office to document my last review when I saw a new message in my inbox.

It was from intensive care and related to a woman in her fifties who had been found at home with an unrecordably low blood sugar following what looked like an accidental insulin overdose. She had been lying there for some time, and although she was alive she was profoundly unconscious. Her CT brain scan showed signs of a severe metabolic brain injury, presumably a result of prolonged hypoglycaemia and low oxygen levels. She had by now been on ICU for two weeks and was off all sedative drugs but she remained unresponsive: her conscious level was four out of fifteen (three is the lowest score) and was not changing. Could I please come to assess the patient and speak to her family about prognosis? I looked at a few recent notes entries. The ICU consultant felt there was no chance of her recovering consciousness and had suggested withdrawing life-supporting treatment, but her family had objected. The patient's son was a corporate lawyer in the US and was now on the unit accusing the hospital of trying to murder his mother.

This did not sound like the kind of consultation you could fit in between a multiple sclerosis relapse and a migraine. To add a rushed interaction with an overstretched neurologist into a highly charged situation would be like throwing a lit match into a gas leak. I was being stitched up like a kipper and felt that this merited at least a phone call from the ICU doctors.

As I considered how best to respond it crossed my mind how very different the experience of a neurologist is now from the older generation of consultants under whom many of us trained. When I started consulting at a general hospital there were fewer neurologists and we were less available. This meant that the medical teams who wanted you to see their patients helped you, lending you a junior doctor to talk through the cases and documenting for you as you went. Rewind further and the experience is even more removed. One of the neurologists in the post-war period (all men then) would arrive for his ward round in a chauffeur-driven Bentley, immaculate in a well-pressed suit, and would sweep up the steps into the entrance hall. Here a line of waiting functionaries would fall into step alongside him as they headed up to see patients who had been tweaked and preened for the great man's arrival.

Now, consultants respond to relentless electronic requests as if we are delivering takeaways, trawling about the wards on our own, deciphering notes and taking a series of decisions under pressure. The vision in a suit is no more – we are more likely to cut a harried and slightly dishevelled figure, with cycling trouser clips sitting forgotten above comfortable shoes and clutching a bag stuffed with papers. If your review is 'discharge-dependent' then you might get a phone call from one of the managers asking you to hurry up.

I got hold of the ICU consultant on the phone. He was apologetic for the cursory referral and told me that in fact my input was no longer needed. The lady's condition had deteriorated as her brain had swollen up and she had succumbed that morning. The staff on the unit were doing their best to comfort her family.

The extent of this lady's brain injury had been catastrophic. Often, though, people will survive even severe damage, as Anton did after a prolonged cardiac arrest or, alternatively, following severe trauma or stroke. Once the patient is stabilised the question inevitably arises: are they going to wake up? It is a common request for neurologists to come and make this assessment on an ICU.

The scenario which we absolutely must not miss here is locked-in syndrome, which occurs when somebody has damage to the front of their pons – usually from a stroke – that completely disconnects all descending motor tracts from the body. The patient is fully awake and yet no commands can leave their brain's hemispheres: the result is complete paralysis of their limbs, face and speech. To the casual observer the patient appears entirely unresponsive but a closer look soon reveals that this is not the case. Eye movements are typically spared and remain connected to the cerebral hemispheres, forming the only link through which the patient can potentially communicate with the outside world.

Once this syndrome is recognised and the eye movements are harnessed then communication is possible and the patient can exert a degree of control over their surroundings. The French journalist Jean-Dominique Bauby famously 'dictated' an entire book, *The Diving Bell and the Butterfly*, relating his experiences of this condition by blinking his left eye. Over a century before locked-in syndrome was first reported in a medical context Alexandre Dumas described a man with something very similar in *The Count of Monte Cristo*. Monsieur Noirtier had been stricken with what Dumas called apoplexy – he later specifies that this was caused by a burst blood vessel in his brain – which had left him entirely motionless. He was nursed propped up in a chair but 'the speaking eye sufficed for all. He commanded with it; it was the medium through which his thanks were conveyed. In short, his whole appearance produced on the mind the impression of a corpse with living eyes.' Dumas then describes how Noirtier's family used a combination of blinking and a dictionary to help him communicate his thoughts and desires.

Usually in an ICU setting this possibility will already have been ruled out, as will reversible causes of unresponsiveness such as seizures: the cause of the patient's low level of consciousness is extensive brain damage. The question is whether they are aware at all of their surroundings. And if not, is this likely to change?

This assessment is difficult and complex, involving clinical examination, scans and other investigations such as recording brainwaves. Sometimes you can be quite definite as to likely prognosis, but often this is not possible. If there remains a wide range of possible outcomes then it may be that no moves are made to withdraw life-sustaining treatment early on – the patient may be moved from ICU to a regular ward with little to be done but wait. At this point they enter a hinterland of uncertainty.

*

Philip was cycling home from work. It was after midnight and he had just finished a late shift at the supermarket in his local town, setting off on the thirty-minute ride with lights on and reflective gear in place. He was in his early thirties and lived by himself in a small Suffolk village. Home was one valley along from his place of work, and the road he followed was bordered with tall hedges on either side as it rose gently to the dark skyline. The moon had not yet risen. It was a lonely stretch, with no signs of life in the pastures to either side, and as Philip slowly climbed the hill the only sound was a faint rustling from the rooky woods beyond.

Then the silence was broken by the sound of an engine over the brow of the hill, out of sight but gaining fast. The hedgerows lit up. Philip looked up in horror as a blaze of light bore down upon him. The slight curve in the road had brought the speeding van across to his side as it breached the top of the hill. He made a dive for the ditch but not in time. The van's corner caught him hard and at speed – he was catapulted against a tree with violent force.

The paramedics found Philip twenty yards from his wrecked bike. He had obvious injuries and fractures in many parts of his body but the immediate concern was the lack of a pulse – he was in cardiac arrest. Working at the side of the road, they put a tube into his airway and started CPR. Having immobilised Philip's neck and transferred him onto a board they headed at speed for the nearest hospital. While they hurtled down the country roads they made a hole in his chest wall and inserted a drain: now Philip's heart began to respond. By the time they arrived he had a pulse and a recordable blood pressure but was profoundly unconscious.

The list of Philip's injuries stretched to nearly thirty lines on a page and included skull fractures, complex fractures to three of his limbs, several ribs and seven spinal vertebrae. In the first week he needed six orthopaedic operations and insertion of a bolt to measure the pressure in his skull. The coming weeks saw more procedures, including repair to his aorta, further limb surgery and a tracheostomy. His brain injury was severe. There were collections of blood around the hemispheres on either side, contusions within the lobes in several places and MRI evidence of shearing damage to his white matter tracts. Pressure was building up within his brain's ventricles, so he needed insertion of a shunt tube to allow this to drain, but his clinical state was unchanged: Philip remained unconscious.

As the medical dust settled, a picture began to emerge of the effects of Philip's brain injury. There was no movement at all on the right side of his body and spasticity was gradually pulling that arm and leg into a flexed posture. There was some spontaneous though non-purposeful movement in his left arm but only within a limited range. With time Philip began to open his eyes for short periods, and he sometimes tracked people around the room. He showed no ability to obey an instruction nor any attempts to communicate.

There is a difference between being awake and being conscious. If somebody is in a coma then they are neither: their eyes are closed, they have no sleep cycle and show no response to a painful stimulus. After a brain injury of whatever cause, assuming the brainstem is more or less intact, people usually come out of coma fairly quickly. But it is possible to show signs of wakefulness – eyes open during the day but closed at night, grimacing or pulling away in response to a pinch – while remaining entirely unaware of the world around you. These responses are reflex behaviours which depend only on brainstem functions – they require no awareness. This 'unresponsive wakefulness state', also called the 'vegetative state', represents the first rung above coma on what is sometimes called the consciousness ladder.

Philip was certainly awake at times, so was well out of coma. The fact that he sometimes made eye contact suggested that he was to some extent aware of those around him and so was also beyond vegetative. Philip occupied the next rung up the ladder, described as a minimally conscious state, where patients do show reproducible signs of being aware of their environment but these are fleeting and inconsistent. The upper echelon of this category, 'minimally conscious plus', includes some element of language such as following an instruction or trying to speak. For now this was beyond him.

The extent of Philip's injuries, quite apart from brain trauma, meant that he was beset by medical issues which took his energies and attention away from any attempts at therapy. He had a tracheostomy which needed frequent suctioning of secretions and had recurrent chest infections. He would often have episodes of vomiting when being fed through a tube in his stomach. With each medical setback he would become very fatigued and his conscious level would slip a little down the ladder, taking weeks each time to recover, and this cycle went on for months. Despite therapy input Philip remained minimally conscious and entirely dependent. After almost a year he was discharged to a nursing home where the cycle of infections and vomiting continued.

Philip came into our care some time later at a point when the legal process had worked its way through so that there was funding for a no-holds-barred intensive neurorehabilitation admission – this is what we were charged with delivering. He appeared one day in a side-room and I met him with senior speech therapist Seána. As we approached the bed she introduced me.

'Hello, Philip, it's me again, Seána. This is Dr Swayne. He's a neurologist and he'll be your consultant while you're with us.'

Her Dublin accent carried a reassuring weight of experience behind it.

Philip was definitely awake and his eyes were wide open. He looked up and met my gaze for a few seconds, clearly registering my presence, before looking back at Seána. He had delicate, almost childlike features, his eyes set like limpets beneath a large domed forehead, and his face was pink and shiny with a faint sheen of sweat. Intelligent eyes looked out through steel-rimmed glasses and a slight slant to his mouth lent him a quizzical expression. Philip's arms were held bent at the elbows, his wrists were flexed awkwardly and his fingers splayed out like fans. His right arm was fixed and immobile but his left waved about slightly, his only semi-mobile limb. Perched high up on the hospital bed among a sea of pillows, he looked like a crown upon a cushion.

Seána and I tried some yes/no questions – was he at home, was his name Philip, did he have a sister? He looked as if he wanted to answer but somehow the effort involved was too great. There were no attempts to speak but we saw occasional nods of the head, small and brief, and for a while we had a reliable yes answer to a series of questions, before his fatigue kicked in and he closed his eyes. Lying beached on the hospital bed, tracheostomy gurgling slightly, tubes in his tummy and bladder, Philip looked exhausted. He had been in this situation now for over three years.

The first job from my perspective was to achieve a period of medical stability. I engaged an ENT surgeon to optimise his tracheostomy and together with Seána we carefully balanced medications, reducing the burden of secretions that kept going down onto his chest while keeping them loose enough so that he could cough them up when they did. I asked a gastroenterologist to look into the recurrent vomiting. We had a number of orthopaedic surgeons review his many limb issues and we loosened his stiff muscles with targeted Botox injections. We rescanned his brain and asked a neurosurgeon to adjust the shunt system that was draining his ventricles. Meanwhile the therapists got stuck in as best they could but the windows of engagement were very brief.

Some time later we admitted Bridget. She was a wiry and dynamic woman in her late forties, a restless spirit who, while born and raised in the UK, had lived abroad for much of her adult life. Her passion was education and this took her to Sri Lanka, where she ran a charity while her husband Dan worked in a development organisation. The work was demanding and took her all over the country. She and Dan had no children and after five years in Colombo they had developed a heady social scene which filled their spare time with friends and trips around the beautiful Sri Lankan countryside.

Celebrations for the Lunar New Year were in full flow when Bridget had begun to feel unwell in a way that she found hard to define. At first she thought that perhaps she had just been overdoing it. But after a few days she also began to feel wobbly on her feet, taking longer to get about and then needing to hold onto Dan's arm. She was admitted to hospital in Colombo for tests and while there was not herself at all, rambling in conversation and sometimes disorientated. The doctors were concerned about a possible encephalitis but a lumbar puncture found nothing amiss in her spinal fluid and a brain scan was unremarkable. They treated her with anti-viral medication to cover the possibility of infection and waited for her to respond.

Bridget really did not get on with the hospital environment and found the constant supervision oppressive. The doctors suggested that while they waited for some of the tests to come back she could perhaps go home for a day over the weekend, returning to the hospital in the evening. Dan drove her back to their bungalow and held her arm as she slowly climbed out of the car and made her way indoors. The relief was immediate and spirits were high as they ate lunch together but when Bridget went to the bathroom later that afternoon Dan heard a sickening crash. He found her lying flat on her face, blood gushing from her forehead which, it seemed, had struck the side of the basin. Her eyes were open and as Dan turned her over she reached out and held his hand, but she was not speaking and even as he phoned for help she was becoming drowsier.

Bridget was rushed back to the hospital but on the way lost consciousness altogether. By the time she arrived her pupils were not responding to light and a CT scan showed a large collection of blood inside her skull on the left, pushing her brain several centimetres across and downwards. She was rushed to theatre and the blood was drained but the neurosurgeons noted that her brainstem was being pushed hard into the bottom of her skull. Sedation was gradually lightened and then removed but Bridget did not wake up. A week later she was able to breathe for herself and the ICU doctors began to talk about putting in a tracheostomy to protect her airway, but her pupils were still not reacting and she remained unresponsive to any attempts to rouse her. Dan kept a vigil at Bridget's bedside, talking to her and holding her hand, but she lay with her eyes straight ahead and showed no sign that she was aware of his presence. Dan became increasingly desperate at the lack of any progress and as the doctors could give him no signs of hope he began to make arrangements to get her back to the UK. It was around three months after her injury when Bridget arrived at our hospital.

Seána and I knocked and let ourselves into her side-room where we found Dan sitting by her bed reading to her from a newspaper. We shook hands and talked through the events that had led to this point. Dan was fresh-faced and clean shaven, sporting a polo shirt and jeans. He had a measured, easy manner and I warmed to him immediately. Dan told us that in all the time since Bridget had come out of surgery he had not seen her move her arms or legs in a purposeful way, nor move her eyes to meet his gaze. Two weeks previously she had begun to make chewing movements from time to time, and to scrunch her lips up in a grimace, but he did not think that this related to anything he said or did. I asked if he felt that she was aware of his being there. He thought about this.

'It's so hard to know,' he said. 'Sometimes when I come in and say hello I feel that she hears my voice but I can't put my finger on why I think that. She doesn't move or look at me but she seems to become a little more alert somehow. Nothing concrete.'

I examined Bridget while Dan sat and watched. She had a tracheostomy in her neck and was breathing for herself. She lay stock still with her eyes half open and her arms by her sides. I made a loud clap beside one ear and her eyes gave a faint flicker in response. I lifted her lids to find that her eyes were pointing in slightly different directions and she did not flinch when I waved a hand in front of her eyes. Her pupils showed no response to a bright light yet when I moved her head from side to side they remained pointing ahead as they should.

Other reflexes likewise suggested that her brainstem was at least partly working. There was considerable stiffness building up in her limbs: when I gently bent one of her legs it pulled into a strong involuntary spasm, her thighs clamping together and her knees bending. This eased after a few seconds but it did not take much to trigger another leg spasm and she was already on high doses of medication to reduce these. I tried giving a pinch above her eye: after a second or so she grimaced and her arms and legs bent slightly in response. A pinch in the fingers or toes induced the same reaction but she made no movement to pull my hand away.

Dan was quietly positive in his interactions with me, and he said that while he realised Bridget had shown no improvement so far he was sure we would do our best for her. He seemed entirely rational in discussing Bridget's predicament. Putting myself in his shoes, I would have been a gibbering wreck. It was too early on in our assessments at that point to give him a definitive view as to how things were likely to go, but on first review it did not look good. An EEG recording of her brainwaves showed that while these were present, and she had no epilepsy, they were extremely slow. We recorded over the scalp and found that her brain lacked an electrical response to a visual stimulus such as a flash of light but it did respond to a sound. Sensation in her limbs was also getting through.

Initial examinations had showed no evidence that Bridget was aware of her environment but in patients who are in a state of low awareness – known these days as a prolonged disorder of consciousness – small signs can be important and a proper assessment takes longer. We have a number of structured tools for doing this which involve observation and a number of manoeuvres designed to stimulate a response. When we went through all of these Bridget scored very low. Her responses put her in the category of an unresponsive wakefulness state – she was vegetative.

By now it was around four months after her head injury and the longer people remain static the less likely they are to change in the future. We had repeated a range of tests as to the cause of her initial illness – could she perhaps still have an encephalitis? – but we found no signs of anything to explain it and at this point it was likely to remain a mystery. We got her off all sedating medication, replacing the anti-spasm drugs with a pump system that delivered them directly to her spinal cord. Her legs were now nice and loose, but still we saw no change in her awareness.

*

I sat with Dan in a small office just off the ward and we looked together through Bridget's brain scans. I scrolled through the MRI images which showed slices of her head viewed from below and explained what the pictures meant as I worked my way upwards and then back down again. The brain's contours were normal enough, but in many places its usual clean black appearance was sullied with the white smudge of damaged tissue, an extensive pale haze that included wide reaches of the cerebral hemispheres but also parts of the brainstem. The damage was extensive and I explained to Dan that the overall picture was consistent with a scenario in which Bridget would have little or no awareness of the world around her. We still had some tricks up our sleeve – medications that we could try – but at the moment her level of consciousness did not seem to be changing.

Dan had been looking carefully at the images on the screen through a pair of glasses. He now took these off, leaned back in his chair and closed his eyes. I had not seen him show any distress to this point but now as he sat quietly a tear rolled down one cheek. I waited. After a minute he opened his eyes, turned to me and smiled.

'Bridget always wanted an adventure. When we first got together – so long ago now – we realised we wanted the same things from life. See the world, go to far-flung places. Do some amazing things together. So we didn't have kids and we just got on with it. And we did have an adventure. We certainly did that.'

We talked a little about some of the places they had been to, Dan at times half laughing and half crying. He then asked me what I thought it was like being Bridget at the moment. Was she aware of anything? I told him that she was probably aware of very little but that this was only guesswork. From what we could tell she was not suffering at all but beyond this it was impossible to know.

How could we possibly fathom Bridget's experience of being alive? We rely on language to communicate our experience of the world to others, and failing that we have gestures and facial expressions. Even within the horrors of locked-in syndrome the eyes provide a line of communication, however tenuous: a window that allows us to peer into the patient's experience. For somebody in a vegetative state, we have nothing. What is their world like? I sometimes conduct a thought experiment in which I strip away my neurological functions one by one. Speech gone. Vision black. Arms paralysed. Legs immobile. Hearing – not sure. What remains? Am I alone with my thoughts and memories or can I not even access these? I imagine being a disembodied figure floating at the bottom of a dark pond, vaguely aware perhaps that something goes on above the surface but unable to access it.

This is pure fancy of course, but in 2006 something happened which changed how we think about patients in this state. In Cambridge a team of neuroscientists led by Adrian Owen used the relatively new technique of functional MRI scanning to study changes in blood flow within the brain of a woman in her early twenties who showed no outward sign of being conscious. She had suffered a brain injury six months previously in a car crash and ticked all the boxes for being in a vegetative state. They wanted to know whether fMRI scanning might reveal signs of awareness which were undetectable clinically. First they looked for changes in blood flow in response to hearing speech and compared this to the patient's response to acoustically matched meaningless sound. When healthy people hear such phrases they activate language-specialised regions in the temporal lobes and it turned out that this woman responded with a similar pattern of activity. But while this shows that her language network was partly intact it does not necessarily mean that she was conscious. Information from the outside world triggers activity in our brains' sensory processing regions all the time whether we like it or not – a flash of light in our eyes causes the occipital cortex to flare up briefly, for example – but this does not mean that we are aware of it.

She was next given verbal instructions – played over a speaker during scanning – which would require a sustained and deliberate response. In one 'task' she was asked to imagine that she was playing tennis, repeatedly swinging her right arm to hit a ball over the net – an imagery task that in healthy subjects activates a specific frontal motor region. In another she was asked to imagine walking around her own house – a navigation task that usually activates a frontoparietal network.

As the scan went on and the instructions were played the woman showed no outward response. And yet the same brain regions sprang to life as for healthy people: the motor region for the tennis task and the spatial network for the navigation task. This was no brief automatic response – to be detectable in that MRI protocol she must be activating these regions for sustained periods of time. More importantly, unlike the passive listening protocol these tasks involved a degree of active participation: she must be *choosing* to take part in the task. Neuroscientists argued extensively at the time about what this result meant but I can see no reasonable conclusion other than that she was aware of the instructions and decided to comply with them. To some extent at least she was conscious.

This important result was followed four years later by a larger study in which five out of fifty-four patients with prolonged disorders of consciousness could modulate their brain activity in a similar way. This led to the terrifying thought that of the thousands of people around the world who were alive but apparently unaware, a proportion may in fact be conscious but unable to show it. The phenomenon of being conscious but with no means of making a physical response has become known as cognitive-motor dissociation (CMD) or covert awareness.

A functional MRI scan is a long and unwieldy process which makes it an awkward tool to look for covert awareness more widely. More recently a Chinese group have developed a clever technique which uses EEG electrodes over the scalp to record the brain's electrical fields while the patient is shown two images side by side. The patient is asked to focus their attention on one of them and a computer interprets the brainwaves to determine which side they are attending to. If they can do this correctly with a degree of consistency which is beyond chance then that patient is deemed to be following the instruction, and to be covertly aware. If this technique is applied early on after a brain injury it appears to have some use in predicting which patients are likely to regain consciousness over the coming months. A larger study in 2024 used either the fMRI or the EEG technique in over three hundred patients with severe brain injury who could show no physical response to an instruction: by these criteria a quarter of these patients showed covert awareness.

This finding unquestionably changes how we might approach somebody like Bridget. She had unfortunately shown no significant change over several months despite all that we could throw at her. Her eyes remained half open and fixed straight ahead, unresponsive to any stimuli. She made chewing and grimacing movements and these were a little more prominent if she was in a position of discomfort but otherwise did not obviously relate to the outside world. Dan was in the process of moving back to the UK so was coming and going but he video-called her every day and talked her through whatever had been going on while a nurse held the phone up in front of her eyes. Bridget's sister also called often and her old friend Jean visited and read her stories. Jean reported that on two occasions while she was reading to her Bridget had appeared to shed tears, though it was hard to be sure that this was connected to what she was hearing.

We were keen to look for evidence of covert awareness in Bridget but the neuroscience techniques involved are not routinely available. We managed eventually to arrange this as part of a research study and some months after Bridget's injury one of Adrian Owen's collaborators studied her responses to the standard tennis task. Her arms were secured at her side by a blanket and she was slid across from her trolley onto the MRI table. Once all of the electrodes were in place and we had a good signal on her pulse and oxygen levels she was slid slowly into the belly of the machine, her head disappearing into the scanner's cold metal tunnel. We peered through the glass screen from the control booth where the radiographer started the scanning protocols: the machine settled into an intermittent high-pitched drone, somewhere between a circular saw and a car alarm. I listened in on Bridget's headphones from which a calm female voice was instructing her when to imagine swinging a tennis racket and when to rest. If she minded the noise and discomfort she did not show it – she stared serenely upwards as before. Lying inert and dignified as the noise swirled around her, she reminded me of the bronze effigy of a Plantagenet queen.

Bridget completed the tennis task five times and on two of these there was activity in one of the relevant motor regions. On the other three occasions, though, there was no such pattern and none of the EEG recordings showed any response to the task. The conclusion was 'possible CMD'. So what should we make of this? Was Bridget aware or not? It is important to recognise the limitations of what these changes on a scan can tell us. For a start, in the largest study to date only around two-fifths of those patients who could outwardly follow an instruction could in fact modulate their brain activity to command. Presumably then damage to the brain's networks affects different kinds of response differently. More importantly, perhaps, we need to consider what the ability to follow such an instruction might mean for somebody's experience of life. What is required for us to be aware of the world around us?

Before we can be conscious we must first be awake. Coma may have many causes – brain injuries, strokes, drugs, a general anaesthetic – but all of these have in common a greatly reduced degree of activity in neurons right across the cerebral cortex. Usually, cortical activity is supported from below by the reticular activating system, a network of upward projections from the brainstem that fan out and promote synaptic activity. When this network is damaged directly this support is lost: the cortex's neurons become unexcitable and the EEG recording of brainwaves is slow and flat. It is hard to imagine any sort of awareness being present in such a brain. But in the vegetative state patients appear to be unaware despite this arousal network remaining intact, and sometimes have relatively normal rhythms on EEG. Are there specific brain regions that must be preserved in order for consciousness to be supported?

Much as in the language and visual systems, it seems increasingly that it is the integrity of networks rather than specific regions which is important. Two networks in particular seem to play key roles: the anterior forebrain mesocircuit – a series of connections between regions near the brain's centre – and a frontoparietal network. The arousal pathway coming up from the brainstem feeds into these networks, and in those patients who do gradually climb back up the consciousness ladder these connections seem to come back to life.

Insertion of a long, thin electrode directly into the central thalamus – similar in principle to the deep brain stimulation now used commonly in Parkinson's disease – has improved alertness in a small number of patients with severe brain injury, but the changes were modest. Electrical or magnetic stimulation of the brain's cortex may support alertness to a degree, but again, they do not seem to be transformative. Medications can support these ascending networks and many have been tried, but only one has any proven benefit – an anti-viral drug called Amantadine which boosts dopamine levels – and again this is not usually dramatic. We had given careful trials of three such medications to Bridget but had seen little if any change.

If somebody shows a positive MRI response to the tennis task they must presumably be able to integrate information across remaining networks sufficiently that they can hear an instruction, understand it and initiate a thought process. But this still does not tell us what their conscious experience is like. To what extent is what they are doing automatic? The brain offers many examples, such as blindsight, of the difference between perception and awareness – we can only speculate as to whether brain activity reaches a conscious threshold.

The usual definition of being conscious is having a subjective experience. The nature of the link between the brain's physical processes and what we experience is often called the 'hard problem' of consciousness and this means different things to different people. To some it is a non-problem – our subjective experience is simply the sum of the neural activity in our brain and 'consciousness' as such is a philosopher's construct. Others feel that something else is needed to bridge the perceived gap and, depending on who you are, this could be a spiritual soul or something else. There is indisputably a point where we come up against the limits of science's descriptive powers: the question perhaps is how important you feel this gap is in attempts to explain our subjective experience.

If you put the hard problem to one side and try to describe subjective experience in purely neuronal terms, then what remains is still not exactly easy. One elegant way of looking into this is the binocular rivalry paradigm, where a healthy subject is presented with a different image in each eye – a house in one and a face in the other – such that they overlap. We can deliberately shift the spotlight of our attention according to what we decide to focus on. If we are asked a question about the house then activity surges in our parahippocampal gyrus (the place region). If instead we need to focus on the face then activity shifts to our fusiform gyrus (the face region). So brain activity moves about according to what we are attending to, engaging relevant networks according to the nature of what is under consideration.

There are a number of models of what we are doing when we are keeping something in our mind's eye. One popular model sees our conscious experience at any given moment as arising from a 'global neuronal workspace', a widely distributed network of cortical regions acting as a sort of mental buffer to hold a piece of information or a perception temporarily in a form that we can use for something. Our working memory should be part of such a workspace and is known to depend on frontoparietal networks – since damage to these causes reduced awareness, this seems a promising model.

From Bridget's scans it was clear that she had damage to several of these networks. She could sometimes respond to the tennis task, but at other times she could not – to me this suggests that her ability to fire up the injured connections between remote brain regions varied depending on her overall state of arousal. Likewise one might imagine that a brain network which is fragmented by injury might support a degree of awareness at some times but not at others. In my simple view of lying beneath the surface of a pond I think of such patients as bobbing slowly up and down, at times far out of reach in the murky depths and at others nearer the surface and the world beyond the water.

Family members of patients in low awareness states will often report behaviours that the clinical team may not see or do not recognise as evidence of awareness. Bridget had twice shed tears while being read to: was she emotionally moved by what she heard or was it a physical reflex? The nurses and therapists had witnessed occasional tears in other contexts, but perhaps she was moved then too. For understandable reasons family may want to read awareness into what is in fact reflex behaviour or imbue a facial expression with emotional content that is not real. But, equally, who is to say that at times this is not the case? It makes sense to me that islands of conscious behaviour may emerge from time to time.

Derick Wade, a neurorehabilitation professor who has worked for many years with patients in low awareness states, has described treating a farmer who after an acquired brain injury had remained in a vegetative state and shown nothing approaching complex behaviour for more than four years. As a group of friends stood around his bedside one day one asked another to remind him what those white ducks were called. The supposedly unconscious patient piped up quite clearly: 'Aylesbury duck.' He then sank back into the depths of unawareness.

If patients in prolonged disorders of consciousness can fluctuate to such a degree then one might argue that terms such as vegetative state or minimally conscious state are too concrete. The very word 'state' implies stasis. But while such moments of awareness may yet be present they are very often fleeting and it may still be the case for many that the majority of their experience is far removed from ours.

A patient such as Bridget depends for nutrition and hydration on liquid feed provided through a tube into their stomach. From a legal perspective this is described as 'clinically assisted nutrition and hydration' and it is considered to be an active medical treatment. In 1993 the UK courts considered the case of a man in a vegetative state which, according to expert advice, was felt to be permanent. The judge ruled that as this patient would always remain unaware the continued provision of nutrition and hydration was a futile medical procedure from which he derived no benefit. The medical team were therefore entitled to withdraw this treatment, from which the man's death inevitably followed, and the precedent was set for such a process in patients with no chance of recovery. This applied to patients in a 'permanent vegetative state' but since we now recognise that such categories may be less rigid than previously thought the process for making such decisions has moved towards a 'best interests' approach. Very rarely somebody will have made a written advance directive stating their wishes for such a situation but this is not usually the case. Since we cannot ask the patient's opinion on their future we need to consider very carefully what they would want to do if they were able to make such a decision themselves.

These are inevitably difficult discussions. The clinical team needs to provide an estimate of what that person's overall quality of life is likely to be and how things may evolve with time. The family and any significant others will provide a sense of that person's previously expressed opinions and values – have they ever stated previously what they would want in such a scenario? – and then all will consider the key question: are they likely to lead a life that they would value? Often there is a clear consensus but opinions may vary and when a joint position cannot be reached then the decision will be referred to the court of protection.

A few considerations make discussions about withdrawal of treatment even harder than they would be already. One is the inability to give absolute certainty as to the long-term outcome. Of course nobody can ever be one hundred per cent definite about any future outcome. You can only say in good faith that you are as certain as you can be that somebody will not improve significantly, but you cannot discount the apparent miracle recoveries: a very small number of people have in fact emerged from a vegetative state even a year or more down the line. It is important to remember, though, that even if such a person begins to follow instructions or communicate they are likely to remain profoundly disabled.

The other important consideration is what is sometimes called the disability paradox. This is the observation that healthy people (including healthcare workers) consistently underestimate the quality of life of those with severe disabilities. Put another way, the judgements that healthy people make about whether they would value a life with disability are often very different from what people actually think once the proverbial shit has hit the fan. American psychiatrist James Hall had written an advance directive stating that he would not wish to survive if disabled.

But when he found himself with locked-in syndrome from a stroke he painstakingly used his eyes and an alphabet chart to spell out the words I – D – E – M – A – N – D – T – O – L – I – V – E – A – S – S – H – O – L – E.

This phenomenon is recognised more generally. The biggest quality-of-life survey in locked-in patients to date is a Belgian study – admittedly open to potential selection bias by virtue of being collected through a patient interest group – which received detailed replies from sixty-five such patients who were an average of eight years into their illness. Despite severe ongoing disability 72 per cent declared themselves to be happy. The majority lived at home with their families, and while almost half had at some point in their illness wanted to die, in fact just 13 per cent were depressed.

This 'happy majority' is perhaps a surprising finding in what is often considered a grim neurological state. Yet similar findings are seen in surveys of severe stroke and traumatic brain injury. An Australian study examined outcomes following surgery for traumatic brain injury and focused on twenty patients who had survived for at least three years with what was categorised as severe disability. Most reported near-normal quality-of-life scores for general and mental health. By contrast, when healthcare workers are asked how acceptable they would expect to find survival with severe disability, the answer is usually not at all.

As an able-bodied person it seems hard to envisage reporting a decent quality of life in the face of such loss of autonomy. To make peace with such a restricted set of circumstances must involve relinquishing a whole set of aspirations and desires that will never be fulfilled: from the able-bodied side of the fence the prospect seems unbearable. But at least a proportion of people go through this change and still report satisfaction with life, and this suggests that we are capable of making an internal shift in our criteria for happiness. One might argue that this is no more satisfactory than making do with a poor set of options, like a spouse who stays within an abusive relationship. On the other hand, it may be that people refocus their priorities and sources of pleasure, for example away from work and towards relationships with those immediately around them.

Low awareness states are a different proposition from locked-in syndrome in that, as things stand, we can only speculate as to the lived experience of those affected. Some studies offer possible clues. One patient in a minimally conscious state following brain injury was scanned while watching a suspenseful Alfred Hitchcock film and showed activity in visual regions and frontoparietal networks. This fluctuated over the course of the film in a way that was synchronised with healthy subjects watching the same film, suggesting that the patient may be able to follow the plot in the same way. Another study reported subtle muscle responses around the mouth in response to a series of jokes. This was interpreted as evidence of humour in that patient, who was described as being in a vegetative state following a cardiac arrest.

Reports of this kind are largely single case studies, and as yet we have little idea whether such glimmers of consciousness are to be found more widely or are rarities. It is also not possible to generalise about this patient group who have a wide range of brain injuries: we had clear evidence, for example, that Bridget lacked vision. But we must acknowledge the possibility that a proportion of patients in such states may have internal cognitive processes that are similar, at least in part, to those of fully conscious people. We should also as healthcare professionals have the humility to admit the possibility that responses observed only by family members may at times have genuine emotional content and are not always reflexive.

So where does this leave us when considering whether or not it is in a patient's best interests to continue being fed? As things stand, we cannot reliably ask the patient what they would like to do. When we ask a conscious patient with cognitive impairment what they think about a treatment option we are obliged by law to perform an assessment of their mental capacity to understand the decision. This may be straightforward if the decision is whether or not to have a cup of tea, but consideration of stopping life-sustaining treatment would require a discussion that at present is far from possible. So the decision rests with the clinical team. This is an emotive subject which can provoke heated debates between clinicians who often have wildly divergent viewpoints. For some, this is a field of study that is gradually peeling open the experience of a neglected patient group – the burden of proof rests with clinicians to demonstrate that somebody no longer wants to survive before withdrawing treatment. For others, covert awareness as suggested by a scan or EEG represents the flickering embers of a severely damaged system and implies nothing approaching a life that most would value.

Withdrawing treatment from somebody is sometimes seen by their family as giving up on them, but it is crucial to keep the patient at the centre of the decision: we must make sure we are treating the patient and not the family. The worst option is not to discuss it at all, and this happens too often. Bridget had shown subtle changes in her responses, particularly to her family, and discussing her treatment in hospital we felt that it was too early just then to be certain of her trajectory. She was moved to a specialised centre where her family could visit her often and spend time with her.

*

Philip meanwhile was beginning to settle into his routine of therapy and was much more medically stable. He had not had a chest infection for months and was no longer vomiting. The therapists had got him his own chair that was fitted to his particular shape and, thanks to a combination of splints to both elbows and Botox injections, he could now sit out comfortably for hours at a time. As we withdrew some sedating medications Philip became a little more alert and he began sometimes to use his left elbow to indicate yes or no in response to a question. We saw no actual words, though, and his swallowing and airway were still too vulnerable to remove his tracheostomy. We started him on the dopamine-boosting medication Amantadine, and slowly increased the dose.

Philip's occupational therapist was Helen, mid-twenties with large kind eyes, a cascade of blonde curls and a soft Essex accent. She had become very fond of Philip, having worked with him throughout the many months of his admission. One morning she told me that she had a surprise for me and took me into his room. Philip was sitting in his chair watching aviation videos on YouTube – planes were his obsession. Once the video had finished Helen put the tablet to one side and greeted him, asking him how he was today. Having chatted to Philip countless times I was not expecting a response beyond perhaps a small nod, so when he mouthed 'OK' I stopped short. Helen asked him what his mother's name was and when Philip slowly but clearly mouthed the word Jo-se-phine my jaw hung open. She then asked him to spell out his own name and he carefully replied using the phonetic alphabet: Papa–Hotel–India–Lima–India–Papa. At this point I had to sit down.

When Philip had arrived he fell into the category of 'minimally conscious minus', with no evidence of language. Now he was speaking – he had clearly emerged from a prolonged disorder of consciousness. He was more than four years post-brain injury, so we were well out of the period of natural neuronal recovery and from a structural point of view his brain would be entirely static. But we had been pushing hard with therapy, driving his residual capacity for neuroplasticity, optimising him medically and removing obstacles along the way. My view is that having done all this, the addition of Amantadine had been the final step which fired up his remaining networks sufficiently to achieve speech.

Philip continued to fluctuate and when he was tired he would revert to using his elbow – some days he was just not in the mood. But he was much more present than he had been previously and could interact more with those around him. Over the months we were doing this work his family had bought a small bungalow for him, near to his mother and sister so that they could see him regularly. Together with his case manager we orchestrated a complicated discharge to his own home that included twenty-four-hour nursing care, regular input from therapists and a programme of activities.

Almost four years after his injury, Philip was heading back out into the world.

CHAPTER TWELVE

ALL THE KING'S HORSES

Humpty Dumpty never stood a chance. Not only were the thousands of shell fragments next to impossible to piece together but, as far as we know, he never had the attention of a good multidisciplinary team. In neurorehabilitation we have a major advantage over him in the materials we work with – unlike a brittle shell, the brain has some intrinsic capacity for self-repair (natural recovery) and responds to intensive training (neuroplasticity). But even if by some miracle of engineering Humpty's shards could be scraped off the floor, and each one stuck back exactly where it came from, he would still not look quite the same. He would always be slightly different from before he made the ill-fated decision to sit on that damned wall. So who is he now? Is he the same in essence as he was, with only superficial cracks? Is he a scrambled version of the old Humpty? Or is he another egg altogether?

From the wide variety of symptoms to which a brain injury can give rise it would seem that as people we are constructs. The sense we have of ourself as an indivisible whole is a clever artifice, a sleight-of-hand trick our brains perform which allows us to make sense of an otherwise perplexing reality – that we are an assembly of many interacting systems. The modular way in which our many functions are parcelled out – movement, planning, balance, attention, visual perception, emotional control, memory, initiation, empathy – means that a brain injury may leave some intact but others changed or broken. This leaves people somewhat altered and somewhat the same: part of our challenge is to help people adjust to this change and to live the best lives they possibly can in their altered state.

Quite apart from any injury to the brain's structure, the very process of coming through a severe illness has a profound effect on many people which should not be underestimated. A brush with death can profoundly shake anybody's confidence and reset their perspective, a fact that is too often overlooked.

Some years ago I was in Italy with my family when I awoke one morning to a text message from my father. *I don't want to alarm you,* he said, *but I had some sort of collapse yesterday. Apparently there is a split in my aorta and a blood clot sticking into my heart. I don't want to spoil your holiday but I thought you would want to know.* Within fifteen minutes I was in a taxi heading to the airport, my head reeling and my brain switching back into medical mode. As the car climbed up the mountain pass I dialled his number, not knowing quite what to expect, and got straight through. He seemed at once a world away and immediately present, the odd intimacy of serious illness cutting through the distance and the horror.

My father had been rehearsing an amateur orchestra in a church when with no warning he felt faint. He stopped conducting and sank gracefully to the floor but, having done so, made to get up again and carry on. At this point a member of the string section, a retired GP, sat on him and forbade him to move. She called an ambulance and the paramedics found that his blood pressure was worryingly low (the technical term is 'in his boots') so whisked him away to the local hospital. There, an astute junior doctor found differing blood pressures in his two arms – the cardinal sign of a dissecting aortic aneurysm – and performed the correct scan. The lining of his aortic arch, the largest artery in the body which carries all the blood coming out of the heart, had come away and begun to split. Fortunately a blood clot had formed, which had stabilised the situation. Had he stood up again this would not have happened, so the GP had almost certainly saved his life. He needed open heart surgery to replace the entire top of his aorta with a synthetic graft, and for this he would be moved to a specialist cardiothoracic centre. They had kept him flat overnight and were hoping that the clot would remain in place long enough to get him to surgery.

As he told me this I could hear a siren faintly in the background – he was in the back of an ambulance being blue-lighted at speed down a motorway. My mouth was dry as I vaguely recalled that around 50 per cent of patients with ascending aortic dissections do not make it to hospital. As the sawtooth Alps rushed past I sat in a bubble of surreal stasis in the back of my taxi, listening to my father's small voice at the other end and wondering if I would ever hear it again. Decades of overdue conversations compressed hopelessly into half an hour before I had to switch my phone off. On the plane I felt sick.

I was at the hospital by lunchtime, having had good flight luck, but with the pre-op tests he was having and limited access to the ward I only managed to snatch a few minutes with him. He was for surgery the following day. The doctors took time to speak to me and their communication was excellent but, despite the familiar medical setting, there was no doubt that I was now on the other side. In my head I replayed conversations I had had with families of critically ill patients over the years. I hoped I had done a good job.

Back at my dad's house the following day, my stepmother and I dug asparagus beds and hung about while we waited for a call. It was an eight-hour-plus operation. For much of this time his entire body's circulation would be on a bypass machine, the arteries to his brain disconnected completely and temporarily replumbed while the surgical team painstakingly sewed in the aortic graft. Even setting aside the immediate risks of such a major operation, what was the chance that he would be unaffected?

The surgeon called: all had gone smoothly and my father was as well as could be expected at this point. He was beginning to wake up and there were no signs of stroke or any other complication as far as they could tell. He would remain on the ICU for now and, if all was well, would move to the ward in a few days. Barring a bit of ICU-related delirium (he sent me a few text messages in the night: *You have to get me out of here. They are using the intensive care as some sort of knocking shop – there's a couple at it in the next bed!*) he was soon lucid and cheerful, if a bit sore. In fact he was rather relishing all the attention.

We got him home about ten days later, driving slowly so as to avoid bumps which he felt sharply in his split sternum, and sank him gently into a hot bath. I sat and chatted to him while he soaked and, as I did, I thought he looked tired but fine. I wondered at the miracle of being able to replace somebody's entire aorta in less time than it took the internet company to replace our router. He was achy and slow for weeks afterwards but, as the physical effects of this assault slowly waned, he began to get outdoors again. I would have loved to have seen the surgeon's face at the follow-up appointment when my father told him he had been splitting logs with an axe ('*You do know you are on blood thinners, Mr Swayne?*').

But as the physical effects of my father's illness retreated this progress was not matched initially by a return to musical activities. There was crushing fatigue and disabling spells of dizziness, a hangover from the migraines of his youth. Most of all, though, he felt cognitively slowed, as if his thought processes were mired in treacle. Cognitive change after heart bypass is definitely a thing – probably due to tiny fragments of blood clot heading up into the brain – so this was feasible, but to my eyes there was no objective change. To me he seemed as sharp as ever and while recovering had even written over a hundred sonnets. And yet on slower days he mooched about not managing to complete routine admin, let alone get any work done.

For a few months this state of affairs did not seem to be shifting. I began to wonder whether perhaps his illness had somehow accelerated the ageing process. After all, we are familiar with the creep of cognitive change that accompanies later life for many, though intriguingly not all: increased fussing and anxiety, a blunting of empathy, a loss of confidence. Whether it is the accumulation of proteins or the furring-up of small blood vessels, the advance of age does silt up the works for many. This process must chip away at the brain networks that make us who we are, so perhaps we could view ageing itself as a slow and protracted brain injury of sorts. Was this what I was seeing? But after six months or so my father slowly surfaced and before too long all cylinders were firing again, at least from my perspective. His brain seemed fine, but the physical illness had brought with it a psychological jolt from which it took a long time and much effort to recover. He admitted that while of course he had a new lease of life he did now feel in some way 'provisional', and this took some getting used to.

*

After a definite brain injury, the change to somebody's identity is more obvious, but even then it can be hard to define. When Philip's bicycle was hit by the speeding van his life was unquestionably and violently changed. Having emerged slowly from a minimally conscious state he was still left with severe disability: a tracheostomy in his neck, only one moving limb, altered cognition and needing a great effort to communicate. While Philip now lives in his own house in his native Suffolk, he depends on a team of skilled people to look after him every hour of the day and night. It might be hard to imagine that much of pre-injury Philip has survived this process, but on speaking to his family they are not so sure. His sister Ellie sees frequent glimpses of 'core Philip' and when I asked her what this was, she had to think about it.

'I am his little sister,' she said, 'and growing up he always liked to be a wind-up merchant. He would call me Shrimp or use my full name – Eleanor – which nobody ever used unless I was being told off. He still does this. I think he thinks it's funny.'

Fatigue remains a large factor in how much Philip is able to do and interact. On a tired day he can barely communicate at all, but if he has slept well then he will be more actively present. Even before his injury Philip was a man of few words, prone to monosyllabic replies unless you were discussing something close to his heart. If the subject turned to planes, science fiction or computers he would light up. This is still the case, according to Ellie. While sitting with him she was fiddling with his model of the Concorde aeroplane and absent-mindedly trying to straighten out its bent nose-cone. Philip had been quiet but at this he became animated and was making a great effort to tell her something. He slowly mouthed the words:

'It – is – supposed – to – be – like – that!'

The family held a birthday party for their mother at Philip's house. Beforehand Ellie had helped Philip choose a birthday card for her and then asked what he wanted her to write on it. His sign-off 'From Philip' seems a little spartan perhaps, but is consistent with what he would have written before the injury. But whereas he would previously have picked an incongruous card as a joke, he now went for a soppier option. When Ellie put one kiss at the bottom Philip became quite agitated and insisted that she add some more. Evidence, Ellie feels, that they are now seeing a more sentimental side to Philip's personality than before. In some ways he is also more proactive than previously. Before the injury he would be quite content to sit at home and watch TV of an afternoon but now, when he has more energy, he insists to his carer that they put on music or go outside. At his request he is taken to a favourite cafe next to an airfield and, as he watches the planes take off and land, Ellie sees real joy in his face.

We can speculate that Philip is finding some pleasure and even fulfilment in the reduced scope within which he now operates. This is necessarily limited, however, and given his level of disability there seems little possibility of future independence or work. But for Thomas – the vicar-philosopher who bled within his brainstem – work was central to who he was. Though his brain injury was less severe than Philip's, when he left hospital he was still having to contend with a significant degree of disability. He could get about indoors using a powered wheelchair but he still needed a lot of help getting in and out of it, and he could not get washed or dressed by himself. He could speak in short, slurred bursts but it took a lot of effort, and when he was tired he was at times hard to understand. And yet he was determined not to let what had happened keep him from his ministry.

Three years down the line, I asked Thomas and his wife Gail how this return to work had gone. It had taken a few months to settle into being at home and the reality of life with a disability, but then Thomas began to itch to get back out into his parish. It was a sober moment when he pulled his wheelchair up in front of the church where this had all started. The chestnut trees now back in full leaf, he looked up at the familiar building and considered how much had changed. Using an appropriately named pulpit frame, and with the support of three people, Thomas could make his way slowly down the church's aisle. He would stand at his frame and address the congregation for short periods at a time. He had always memorised his sermons anyway – the printed copy was really for back-up – but if he needed to read out prayers or other passages then Gail would hold up sheets of paper with enlarged text.

It was very hard work.

Thomas gradually returned to taking services, with a lot of support from colleagues and congregants, but at the end of the day he was exhausted. Other aspects of his role were even harder. Home visits were rarely feasible unless there happened to be a wheelchair-accessible door, and leading meetings would be slow and laborious. They soldiered on for a year but Thomas gradually realised that it was too much. He reluctantly withdrew from his role and began instead to be more active online, where he blogged prolifically on the issues of the day. Thomas and Gail decided to relocate to Bristol, where they had a circle of friends. They bought a fully adapted flat and gradually established a new life there.

Thomas told me that he felt he was still the same person. He had lost his work, but he was now plugged into the church community in Bristol and still took the odd service there. He had a demanding routine of physio and exercises, but this still left him plenty of time to see friends and he had joined a circle of ex-colleagues who got together and played board games. He would still get tired at the end of a day, but he was able to enjoy his renascent social life. Some days he would feel the weight of his disability – the same active mind trapped in a partly broken body – and this would get him down, but then he would remember all the good things he still had. From Gail's perspective Thomas was largely unchanged. He was perhaps missing a filter – the odd risqué joke might slip out – but on balance she felt that he was more patient and in fact happier than he had been before the bleed. Perhaps, she thought, this was because he was less absorbed in work and better able to focus on what was important.

Gail had, I felt, come gradually to this accommodation with a slightly different Thomas. When somebody is cognitively changed after a brain injury their family may sometimes go through a grieving process for the person they knew. This shift may be harder to make if the changes are more cognitive than physical. To see somebody who is deeply familiar in appearance but changed in their behaviour and responses is for some families quite disturbing. It is similar to what Freud called the uncanny, a cognitive dissonance between familiar and unfamiliar which is why dolls are creepy (and why I will never let any robotic carers near me).

Despite cognitive changes we are sometimes told by families that their relative's centre remains unchanged. They may think and behave differently, but at some core level they are felt to be the same person they were beforehand. So what is this unchanged essence and where does it reside? Some feel that this perceived constancy lives only in the eyes of the family, who do not want to see a change: a form of wishful social cognition, perhaps, love altering not when it alteration finds.

But I think there is something to it. At the very end of my mother's life she was cognitively changed. She had severe emphysema from a lifetime of defiant smoking, and having soldiered on regardless as her lungs slowly crumbled she eventually reached a tipping point. Her last three years were a misery of breathlessness, home oxygen and repeated hospital admissions. Over the final months as her body shut down she began to turn in on herself, all of her attention focused on breathing. The cigarettes had narrowed the blood vessels in her brain (I saw the scan) and towards the end she became less engaged, unable to focus and a bit forgetful. The draining away of her vivacity had been gradual but relentless. She had been a whirlwind of a woman. Her small frame would fill a room with warmth, kindness and a legendary if sometimes cruel wit. She was often described affectionately as the rudest woman in Wiltshire.

I sat with her in her cottage a few weeks before she died. She seemed so diminished. Her arms were clamped tightly onto the table's edge (which helps breathing) and her lips pursed with each outward breath. She was hunched like a tiny and furious sparrow, and despite my attempts at chat could not really speak to me for more than a few seconds at a time. At a medical level I felt helpless. As her son I could feel the ground lurch beneath me as I realised how close we were to the end. I was pretty cross with her that she was not going to see my children grow up. Worse still, as she adamantly refused to admit she was dying we could not even talk about it. But despite the sparse conversation, her occasional irritable snaps and the new vagueness, this was definitely still her. The fog would suddenly lift and there would be a brief flash of complete connection.

For half an hour she seemingly ignored me completely while I prattled on with gossip about friends and family. I told her of a funeral I had been to recently where after a long and very Catholic service the guests had walked down a rutted muddy track to the farmhouse for drinks. I joined a stream of locals and Londoners trudging in smart coats and impractical shoes towards the promise of wine. As I did so the actor Joseph Fiennes crawled past me in the same direction in a low silver sports car. He looked like James Bond. But then a rear tyre slipped into the verge and sank into a thick rut: he spent five minutes with spinning wheels before finally making it to the drinks.

As I relayed this non-story my mother turned from the table and fixed me with a wicked smile. 'Ha! Shakespeare in the mud.'

She was in the room again. During these moments the glimpses I got were of the same person, with the same shared jokes and understandings. Families of people with dementia often say the same.

Was I just projecting my mental construct of her onto a shrinking frame? No doubt to some extent, but not entirely. I think it is to do with values and assumptions. Through all the illness and altered thinking, people's values – what they find more or less important – tend in my experience to remain pretty constant. This was certainly true of my mother and I see it also in brain-injured patients.

The family's perspective is important, but one of the greatest rehabilitation challenges (in the true sense) after brain injury is how a patient deals with their own identity change. They may be unable to fulfil their old roles in the same way. They may change overnight from a valued provider and family lynchpin to a passive recipient of care. How they deal with this shift is an important determinant of their future happiness.

Even in healthy ageing the changes can creep up on us, and our mental image of ourselves often lags far behind the reality. In my mind's eye I remain youthful and vigorous. As the hallmarks of age – that stealthy thief – creep into the image I see in my shaving mirror my brain performs a conjuring trick in screening these out. By filling in the salt-and-pepper hair and restoring my hairline to where it was meant to be, my networks of visual perception somehow ensure that I see what I want to see. Until, that is, a threshold is reached and the adjustments they must make become untenable – at which point the illusion slips and the truth dawns. Most of my peers have at some point caught sight of their own reflection in a windowpane and wondered briefly who that stooped and crumpled person might be. In normal ageing at least we get to adjust our sense of who we are gradually – brain-injured people have to make this shift all at once.

For Priya, a teenager at the onset of her encephalitis, the adjustment was even more complicated. As long a time as a year in hospital would feel for most people, it is much longer for somebody on the cusp of adulthood. Dipping her toe tentatively back into the social scene she had left, she found that many of her peers had moved on. Priya could remember all of her time in rehabilitation, including the names of everybody who treated her, but events leading up to that point were hazy and for ICU she had little memory. This is probably no bad thing: some of the fragments of her recollection were frightening. There were epileptic seizures, painful procedures and every sort of indignity imaginable. Once home she felt that none of her friends would understand what she had been through – how could they? A little like a soldier returning from a distant war, she was unsure how she was supposed to feel about who she was now.

Priya's parents were beyond relieved to have her home again and she was soon swept back into family life. But there were unquestionably changes in how Priya was at home. She was quick to lose her temper, getting upset over minor niggles. She was forgetful, not to the extent that somebody needed to watch over her but enough to make a return to college seem daunting. Month by month, though, these issues improved. After being at home for a year she felt confident enough to enrol for a diploma and started working in a nearby theme park, where she soon developed a new social circle. Priya found friendship less complicated with those who had not known her before her illness, and when we met I had the sense that she had almost started afresh. Save for a neat tracheostomy scar there were no outward signs of her ever having been unwell, and I was delighted to see her laugh and joke with the confidence of a mature adult. She was about to apply for a new job and seemed to be looking forward to the future. My mind cast back to early conversations I had had with her parents when it was not yet clear to what extent she would recover. Seeing her again, this was an outcome I would not have dared imagine.

Working with patients like Priya and others over the years, I have been privileged to witness the power of careful multi-disciplinary rehabilitation to transform outcomes and lives after brain injury. Along the way neuroscience has learned so much about the mechanisms of recovery within the brain that we have before us now an array of potential tools by which we might enhance it, opportunities to drive it harder. The research landscape has changed dramatically since as a junior doctor I watched neurosurgical patient Paul fester in his side-room.

And yet. And yet. Somehow it feels as if we are still some way from translating all this knowledge into improved outcomes. The availability of rehabilitation has improved to a degree, but the fundamental therapy that patients receive has not really changed for decades. Taking stroke as the archetypal brain injury, if you look at research funding and healthcare changes, all the action has been at the emergency end of the pipeline with relatively little attention still paid to recovery. Thrombolysis drugs, mechanical thrombectomy, acute stroke units, hemicraniectomies – all of these have improved survival. But despite these advances, around 70 per cent of people with stroke are still left with impairments. There are millions of people who will often live for years following brain injury – they deserve a concerted effort to reduce the burden of disability that at present they still carry. Because of the increased understanding that neuroscience has brought over recent years, there are new avenues to be explored.

The hyper-plasticity and heightened responsiveness to therapy over the first three months or so is a clear opportunity, but our healthcare systems are not set up to capitalise on it. If you are admitted to hospital with a significant stroke the first weeks are dominated by medical tests, fending off complications and an impetus to get you out of hospital as quickly as possible. Seizing this opportunity is difficult even if a concerted effort is being made to maximise early impairment-targeted therapy. In a recent such study at Johns Hopkins in Baltimore the patients spent a third of their waking time alone in bed doing nothing. If we are to be more ambitious in what we are trying to achieve, aiming not just to manage disability but to reduce the impairments themselves, then we probably need to rethink how we go about this.

An existing popular approach involves immobilising the patient's stronger arm in a sling so that they are forced to use the weaker arm. This 'constraint-induced movement therapy' can reduce overall disability but has limitations; for example, the fact that most things we do involve using both hands together. Most importantly, this approach treats the disability rather than the impairment: favouring compensatory movements early on probably impedes the recovery of high-quality movement further down the line.

The hunt is on for innovative ways in which tech might deliver intensive impairment-based training alongside standard therapy. I have tried out some of these new approaches. In one I stood in front of an enormous screen on which I was represented as a dolphin swimming among a shoal of fish. A motion detector tracked the movements of my right arm and, using this as a controller, I swam about the underwater scene catching fish or jumping out of the water. The gestures I needed to make were cleverly designed to improve the quality of my arm movements. In another game I had to flex or extend my fingers inside a glove-like device in order to move a car. Doing well involved moving my fingers individually and opening out my fist, two particularly difficult movements in a post-stroke hand: by doing this thousands of times patients drill these difficult movements until they are easier.

Another gamified therapy would have been perfect for Gary's hemispatial neglect. Wearing a virtual reality headset I was immersed in a colourful and beautiful world in which balloons floated from right to left – I had to track them with my eyes and then catch them using a wand held in my hand, forcing my attention repeatedly to the left side.

While playing these games I felt entirely immersed in the worlds they conjured, and I could imagine how the intense focus they brought might enable patients to shift the impairments they target. It is still unclear whether drilling impairments like this translates into better performance of practical tasks, but when combined with hands-on therapy it seems to offer a good chance of driving change early on.

It may also be that we will work out how to enhance the effects of such training using brain stimulation – magnetic, electrical or otherwise – whether targeting Gary's attention networks, Tarek's language networks or Danny's motor networks. The mixed results of this approach to date may simply reflect the fact that the most effective strategy in a given patient depends on individual factors, such as the precise brain regions affected. Perhaps a more tailored application of brain stimulation may bear fruit.

A group in Pittsburgh published results in 2023 of a study in which they implanted electrodes into the necks of two patients with weak arms after stroke and applied an electrical current to the nerve roots entering the spinal cord. The idea was to make the motor nerves projecting from the cord to the arm more excitable, and so more responsive to the brain's weaker-than-usual motor output. In an analogue stereo system this would be like compensating for a weak signal from a record player by turning the amplifier up higher. The two patients studied showed increased strength, improved reaching movements and better use of the arm. It is not yet clear how widely applicable this approach is but it demonstrates a proof of principle.

But what about those patients with little or no movement on the affected side, in whom the connection between motor cortex and spinal cord has been completely lost? In the late 1990s Austrian neuroscientist Niels Birbaumer demonstrated a brain-computer interface, or BCI, he had developed in which two patients with complete body paralysis due to motor neurone disease were trained to modulate their brain waves to control a cursor. With no movement at all they could 'think' the cursor about the screen and even spell out words: he called this a thought translation device. No invasive surgery was required, only EEG electrodes over the scalp, but the difficulty was that it took hundreds of hours of training and not every patient could successfully make it work. More invasive attempts have been made, electrodes inserted over the brain's surface or even chips with electrodes sticking into the cortex. Impressive movement control has been achieved this way in patients paralysed from stroke or spinal cord injury. But such surgery carries obvious risks, and in some patients implants have ceased to work with time, leaving them with a defunct chip sticking into their brain that cannot safely be removed. These concerns have led researchers to look again at non-invasive BCIs, introducing more sophisticated sensors and applying machine learning to interpret brain activity such that patients can achieve control of a device or even a limb without long and arduous training.

I visited the neuroscientist Surjo Soekedar and his team at their BCI lab in Berlin. We met in the basement of a laboratory wing at the Charite Universitätsmedizin, a sprawling hospital on the banks of the Spree whose halls had been stalked by medical greats of the Victorian era. In his light and tidy office Surjo described their experimental set-up in perfect English, his clipped accent bubbling over occasionally with infectious enthusiasm. He told me they would train patients with stroke to move their weak hand using an exoskeleton operated via electrodes on their scalp: they would then apply this approach to manipulating everyday objects in intensive physio sessions over four weeks.

That morning a new patient was coming in for a familiarisation session and I met her with three of the research fellows in a long, thin lab – workbenches along the sides, stimulators and computers dotted around. In fact, Surjo and I had passed her a little earlier as he showed me around the site: she had been walking slowly towards her appointment with a stick in her right hand and her left arm held flexed. Meeting her, it was confirmed that she was weak on her left side from a stroke in the right thalamus six months earlier, and though she could flex her hand by a few millimetres she could not open out her fist at all. The team sat her in a chair and started by placing a cap on her head into which they placed seven small cylindrical electrodes. This produced an EEG trace on the screen of a laptop, wiggly lines which represented the electrical activity in her motor and sensory cortex. When the team asked her to imagine moving her hand the frequencies in the trace would change. Having analysed this change they made some adjustments and now she was able to open and close the mouth of a Pacman on the screen just by thinking about moving her hand. Her limb remained motionless but the figure on the screen obeyed her will.

Once she could do this with confidence the researchers put her hand into an exoskeleton, a device like a cricket batter's glove but made for Robocop. Each finger was held separately in straps and the whole device connected wirelessly to the laptop. After a few adjustments they switched it on. Her hand had been flexed in a balled-up fist but now, at her mental command, it opened right out, the mechanical servos whirring quietly.

She sat back in her chair with an expression of delighted surprise. 'Ooooh!'

She had not experienced the sensation of controlling her hand since the stroke, and I asked her how it felt. She beamed back at me. 'It feels great!'

In the following sessions the actual training would begin.

Is this simply a fancy splint, a tech-heavy means of achieving the same ends as standard therapy? Probably not, and there is a decent rationale as to how this could help kick-start recovery. When a post-stroke patient uses mental imagery to control an exoskeleton, the physical sensation of the resulting movement arrives in the cortex at the same time as they are trying to generate their own motor output: this closed loop of input and output drives the neuroplasticity needed to remould the motor output. As a result they start to generate small movements of their own – detectable as activity in electrodes over the arm muscles – and soon this itself may be used to drive the exoskeleton and allow further training. By the time the patient has enough activity to make useful movements, the exoskeleton can be removed and the physios can get to work. In this scenario the BCI is being used not just to assist movement but to enhance recovery.

This seems like a great idea but at present it remains just that. If somebody is unable to generate any motor output at all from the affected side then even this approach will have limited potential. Other obstacles include the kit and expertise required, the technical limitations of EEG and the sheer faff of setting it all up each time. But this is changing. Interesting developments are afoot, and it feels like an exciting time to be involved in neurorehabilitation with new treatment avenues opening up. There seems finally to be a chance that some of the neuroscience advances of recent decades may translate into concrete improvements for patients.

*

But even without any new tech, I would settle at the moment for getting the basics right in most people. And at the moment this is often simply not the case. We know two important facts about the 'dose' of therapy people receive after a stroke: first that this is an important determinant of somebody's outcome, and second that what most patients receive is grossly inadequate. There is plenty of evidence for the first of these statements.

Genuinely high-dose, high-intensity therapy programmes are rare beasts, often only seen in the context of research studies, but those for which there is good data perform much better than standard programmes. As to the second statement, to say that patients undergoing 'standard care' rehabilitation do not receive this sort of dose would be a polite understatement. Stroke units in the UK are audited nationally and every working day patients are meant to receive forty-five minutes each of physio, occupational therapy and speech therapy. A 2020 audit found that the median daily dose received in reality were fourteen, thirteen and seven minutes respectively. There are all sorts of reasons why this is the case, including valid logistical difficulties in implementing therapy early on and a lack of resources to make it possible, but the fact is that on stroke units we are under-treating patients during the period they are most sensitive to treatment.

Once patients leave hospital the availability of therapy input is even more scant. We used to be able to pass our patients on to a community therapy team in their local borough to continue the work done in hospital. But austerity economics took an axe to this network, and in many boroughs these teams are thin on the ground. The UK is a patchwork quilt of rehab black holes – once you leave hospital you have largely been cut loose.

The situation in the US is no better, in fact probably worse. A study in 2023 of over seven hundred patients with stroke across twenty-eight hospitals found that by three months over a third had received no physio at all, around half had no occupational therapy and over 60 per cent had no speech therapy input. In the lucky ones who did receive some therapy, the average dose within the Medicare group was a grand total of eleven or twelve hours over the first year. These doses are pitiful in comparison to what we know is required to change impairments – it should be no surprise that a degree of persistent disability after stroke remains the norm.

The argument that proper rehabilitation for stroke and brain injury is a luxury we cannot afford in straitened times does not stand up to scrutiny. Early intensive therapy saves long-term care costs, as it did for Christian. A health economic study including almost six thousand patients having neurorehabilitation across England found that this cost saving was greater in more impaired patients, whose admissions paid for themselves within fourteen months. A similar 2024 analysis for patients with acquired brain injury in Australia calculated that every dollar spent on early rehabilitation saved 91 dollars in the long term.

It is important to emphasise that some brain injuries, including some strokes, are simply too severe for impairments to improve – like Claire, whatever we do the person will unfortunately remain pretty disabled. Even in these patients, though, therapy plays an important role in maximising quality of life. But for many patients, with enough of the right input, the impairments can be shifted and the changes that may be wrought are potentially significant. This is not icing-on-the-cake stuff – for somebody on the cusp of change, such input may mean getting about their own home without help, managing their own affairs or getting out to church on a Sunday. It may be the difference between social isolation and participating in life. It is the best chance they will get to regain the part of themselves that the brain injury has left behind.

So with the knowledge we now have, the high prevalence of disability after brain injury begins to look more like a choice than an inevitability. The people affected are our parents, our peers, our siblings and sometimes even our children. One day it might be you or me. Therapy will only become more available if patients, families and advocacy groups demand it. We should not be accepting a lack of input after discharge from hospital and I would strongly encourage those affected to pester their legislators, insurance companies or local representatives, pointing to the evidence and insisting on better. Having seen patient advocacy groups in action, I would not underestimate their ability to shift public opinion or to apply pressure on those who prioritise resources.

The question of what a country's duty is to its citizens is perhaps one of political philosophy, and in an era of tightening economic restraints discussions of prioritisation become more fraught. But I would argue that if as a society we can afford cars, TV streaming services, holidays and ever smarter computers then we can provide the means for millions living with acquired brain injuries to achieve the best outcomes their conditions allow. To do otherwise makes neither moral nor economic sense.

*

I had been away for a week over the October half term, and was ruddy from Cornish air and round from a surfeit of fish and chips. The spring in my step as I arrived back at work was only slightly diminished after an hour or so in my office going through the usual email deluge followed by a management meeting. I climbed the wide staircase and wandered onto the unit to see what had been going on. As I walked into the day room one of the occupational therapists, Laura, passed me heading fast the other way and spoke to me over her shoulder.

'Welcome back, Orlando, hope you had a good break. So much has happened, lots to tell you! New patient Steve's family have been causing chaos.' She grimaced as she receded down the corridor. 'You've got your work cut out with that one!'

I had no idea yet who new patient Steve was, but I would find out soon enough. Our registrar, Uroosa, was on the phone in the office as I stuck my head in – on hold for the MRI department – and as far as I could tell she had not moved in the week I had been away. I greeted our receptionist, Nefertiti, who was embroiled in a voluble discussion with our rehab assistant Kevin about where the new fire extinguishers should go. As I headed towards the main ward our catering manager was getting involved, brandishing a fish-slice as he spoke. I found our charge nurse, Dennis, in his office on the ward. He was on the phone while working on a staffing spreadsheet and seemed also to have a Teams call on the go. I thought it best not to disturb him but, as he saw me, he stuck his head out of the door.

'Hello, Orlando. No change – the builders are still working on Bay 4!'

He laughed and retreated back into his office, phone tucked under his chin.

My plan was to sit down with Uroosa and catch up on all the medical issues for the ward patients – a paper round – and then to meet some of those admitted while I had been away. She pointed to the phone and rolled her eyes to indicate she was still on hold, so instead I headed to the ward's gym. On my way I passed the therapy kitchen, where I saw Lee standing at the worktop next to a therapist. They were making a nutritious-looking sandwich and as he saw me he nodded.

In the gym the radio was going strong – Heart 80s again – and the plinths were all full. There was a group of patients from the Upper Limb programme in the corner, some doing fiddly things with a therapist while another was working on a robotic arm. Some patients were supine on their plinths as therapists stretched out limbs and strengthened muscle groups, while others were sitting up and working their way through movements. Our neuropsychologist was helping an anxious middle-aged man I did not recognise by distracting him and leading him through mindfulness exercises while he stood up, supported by a physio – maybe this was new patient Steve? As I looked across the busy room I wondered at my luck in working with such extraordinary colleagues, the most consistently kind bunch of people you could hope to assemble.

I had not spotted Patricia, the catering assistant from Essex, who was tucked around the corner from me standing at a pulpit frame, and she brought me out of my reverie.

'Have a nice time off, doctor?'

She was still weak on her right and could not see to that side, but she looked a different person from the confused, hallucinating patient we had received a few months previously. I told her that I had enjoyed it very much, thank you. I always feel a bit guilty going away to some nice place while our patients are stuck in hospital – it seems a little like rubbing salt in the wounds, and I told her so.

'Don't be silly, doctor. We all need a break. I'm spending next weekend at home – have you heard? Hopefully going home for good a couple of weeks after that.'

'I haven't had a chance to catch up about you yet, Patricia, but that's amazing! You've done so well. I should go away more often.'

'I can't wait to get home,' she said. She was quiet for a while then nodded in the direction of the assembled therapists. 'I've got to say, though, I'll miss this lot. They're gold, they are.'

I could not disagree. In my head I congratulated her therapy team, who must have moved mountains to get her home – we had previously thought she might need nursing-home care.

I was brought out of my thoughts by the sound of scraping chairs and people moving plinths to clear a space in the middle of the gym. I asked what was going on and Patricia filled me in. Juliette, our shipping barrister with a stroke, was about to lead a group of patients and staff in a Zumba class. Apparently this was something she did as a stress-busting sideline when she was not in court – now running a class on the unit was one of her rehab goals. As Patricia spoke somebody was already firing up the speaker with Abba and Juliette was limbering up. I started backing quietly out of the door but Patricia caught me.

'Where are you going, doctor? Not going to join us?'

I explained vaguely that I had to go and do some medical bits and pieces with the junior doctor. But Uroosa was at the doorway and she busted me.

'Don't worry, Laura needs me to check some discharge paperwork – I'll be at least ten minutes.'

I was doomed.

ACKNOWLEDGEMENTS

I am immensely grateful to the many patients and their families who agreed to speak to me as I was writing this book. Discussing their experiences will have involved re-living some of the toughest times of their lives. They did so, I know – because they told me – in the hope that promoting wider understanding of the brain's recovery from injury would ultimately contribute to better outcomes for those who may have to go through similar journeys in the future. I would particularly like to thank, in no specific order, Philip and his sister-in-law Sue; Colin and Vicki; Cindy and her sister Tracy; Paul; Lisa; Holly, Jo and Ian; Jesse and Rose; and Nick and Pam.

I have worked over the years with so many wonderful clinicians and scientists that it would be fruitless to try listing them all here, but these are the people who have taught me how to do my job. I would like to single out Richard Greenwood, for his mentorship, wisdom and mischievous dry wit, and John Rothwell for his extraordinary brain. I must thank Leo Cohen for taking a chance on me at the National Institutes of Health, and all of those at the UCL Institute of Neurology who taught me how to do science, at least after a fashion. My many colleagues at the National Hospital – neurologists, neurosurgeons and others – are a dream resource of expertise upon which to draw, and I am lucky to work there. Far from resting on its historical laurels, the National in partnership with the Institute of Neurology continues to discover, to innovate and to improve the lives of patients. May it always continue to do so.

But it is the therapists and nurses I have worked alongside who have really shown me how rehabilitation works. In this respect I am lucky to have found myself among giants: Sarah Daniels, Dennis Minioza – always so patient, whatever the weather – Fran Brander, Kate Kelly, Ronan Burke, Simon Grobler, Lisa Klautke, Celine Lakra and all of the many other colleagues who daily combine great skill with humanity. You are the core of what we all do, and I am so lucky to turn up every day and find you working your magic. I must thank Neesha Galoria, Sabrina Mohammed and Nefertiti Jahaly for keeping the wheels turning, and doing so with consummate grace and humour.

Working on this book has been a great excuse to have many illuminating conversations with expert colleagues and others. I am particularly grateful for comments and thoughts from Becky Burns, Simon Grobler, John Krakauer, John Rothwell, Nick Ward, Alex Leff, Surjo Soekedar, Sara Ajina, Martin Rossor, Jason Warren, Antonio Incisa, Mark Edwards, Diane Playford, Derick Wade, Abi Morgan and my father, Giles Swayne.

The literary process was entirely foreign to me as I embarked on this project. I have been fortunate to be supported through it by wise heads who have not flinched at my naive questions and concerns. Andrea Henry at Picador has been the most thoughtful and supportive editor anyone could wish for, and I must also thank Jessica Yao at WW Norton for her great help. I am very grateful to Chris Wellbelove, my agent, for his honing skills at the proposal stage and for his drive in making it happen. I had helpful early input from Georgia Garrett, Simon Woods and Michael Morris, and crucial advice throughout from Rowan Routh, who is so thoughtful and generous with her time. Without these amazing people there would be no book at all, and I will always be indebted to them.

Finally I must thank the most important people of all: my wife Delia Peel, my daughter Madeleine and my son Sol. Thank you all three for your endless support and encouragement, for putting up with my occasional fits of self-absorption and for being the wonderful people you are. You are the reason I spring out of bed each morning.

REFERENCES

A great many sources have gone into this book, but I would like to highlight the following three as being of particular importance. All are excellent reads, and I have referenced them here extensively.

Friederici, A. D., *Language in Our Brain: The Origins of a Uniquely Human Capacity* (Cambridge, MA: The MIT Press, 2017)

Kolb, B., *Brain Plasticity and Behavior* (Oxford: Taylor & Francis, 2013)

Krakauer, J. W., and S. Thomas Carmichael, *Broken Movement: The Neurobiology of Motor Recovery After Stroke* (Cambridge, MA: The MIT Press, 2017)

In order to spare ink and paper I have not reproduced the full bibliography here, but for those who are interested this can be found at www.howtouseafork.com.